KV-017-841

CONTENTS

CHURCHILL'S POCKETBOOK OF
Obstetrics and Gynaecology

This book is dedicated to Ruth,
Rachel, Ben and Jonathan

For Churchill Livingstone:

Commissioning Editor: Ellen Green
Project Development Manager: Janice Urquhart
Project Manager: Frances Affleck
Design direction: Erik Bigland
Illustrated by: Ian Ramsden

CHURCHILL'S POCKETBOOK OF
Obstetrics and Gynaecology

Brian Magowan

MB ChB DCH MRCOG
Consultant Obstetrician and Gynaecologist,
Borders General Hospital, Melrose, UK

SECOND EDITION

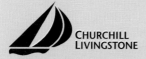

CHURCHILL
LIVINGSTONE

EDINBURGH LONDON NEW YORK PHILADELPHIA
ST LOUIS SYDNEY TORONTO 2000

CHURCHILL LIVINGSTONE
An imprint of Harcourt Publishers Limited

© Harcourt Publishers Limited 2000

🕮 is a registered trade mark of Harcourt
Publishers Limited

The right of Brian Magowan to be identified as
author of this work has been asserted by him in
accordance with the Copyright, Designs and Patents
Act 1988.

First published 1997
Second edition 2000

ISBN 0 443 06423 7
International Student Edition ISBN 0 443 06424 5

British Library Cataloguing in Publication Data
A catalogue record for this book is available from the
British Library.

Library of Congress Cataloging in Publication Data
A catalog record for this book is available from the
Library of Congress.

Medical knowledge is constantly changing. As new
information becomes available, changes in treatment,
procedures, equipment and the use of drugs become
necessary. The author and the publishers have, as far
as it is possible, taken care to ensure that the
information given in this text is accurate and up to
date. However, readers are strongly advised to
confirm that the information, especially with regard
to drug usage, complies with current legislation and
standards of practice.

The
publisher's
policy is to use
**paper manufactured
from sustainable forests**

Printed in China

Contents

Preface to the second edition

There is nothing like updating a broad spectrum textbook written only three years ago to appreciate how much has changed in obstetrics and gynaecology. Not only has the existing text been extensively revised and reorganised, but new areas have been added to include antenatal drug misuse, gynaecological surgery, sexual abuse and legal issues within the specialty. There has been a large expansion both of the chapter on acute obstetrics, with new illustrations, and in the area of prenatal diagnosis, with photographs to clarify the ultrasound perspective.

The aim is to provide an invaluable 'on-the-spot' reference text, not only for medical staff, but also for midwives, medical students and other health professionals. Obstetrics and gynaecology is an intensely practical subject and ownership of this book should not be a substitute for clinical experience. In particular, surgical procedures should be taught on a one-to-one basis under close supervision. In addition, you should never lose the opportunity to see and examine patients and to be involved in the decision-making process for which this book hopes to offer guidance.

Watching parents holding their new baby for the first time is a tremendous experience. It is a privilege to have been involved in some way with a successful birth, and those who have assisted may have feelings of pride and importance. When events go disastrously wrong, however, the feelings of dread and responsibility are often heavy to carry. Parents expect to return home with a healthy baby – they are counting on the doctor and midwife more than on anyone else before, and will remember their care for the rest of their lives.

- As a junior doctor in obstetrics you will probably find yourself calling for seniors' support more often than in any previous post. This is good practice. In addition, do not hesitate to involve other specialists, particularly for medical or surgical problems or with acute labour ward obstetrics.
- Accept that most midwives are more experienced than many junior doctors; listen hard to their opinions.
- When you walk into a labour room, look at the parents before looking at the CTG.
- If you have been involved in a delivery, always see the mother at some stage in her postnatal stay. She will usually be delighted that you took the trouble and it often allows an opportunity to go over what happened.

- Time spent with the bereaved is very important for them and for you. Always allow the family to talk about the one they have lost (use the baby's name if one has been given).
- Beware of amateur scanning.
- Above all, always remember that it is often harder to do nothing than to do something.

Despite the increasing application of scientific techniques, most of obstetric practice carries a large element of uncertainty. Think carefully, however, about how you personally will cope with this uncertainty. Will you become obsessively meticulous, never reassuring your patients for fear of losing your pride? Will you see seek to blame others for your own imperfections? Or will you accept it as the inevitable, but exciting, unpredictability of an uncertain world? It is hoped that this book will provide a practical framework around which to build up a richness of personal experience.

Brian Magowan

Acknowledgements

I would like to thank the following for their painstaking reviews of the manuscript and invaluable suggestions for updating their areas of expertise:

Dr Richard Anderson, Clinical Scientist, Simpson Maternity Memorial Pavilion, Edinburgh – reproductive endocrinology and infertility; **Dr Morag Brown**, Consultant Bacteriologist, Borders General Hospital, Melrose – infection in pregnancy; **Professor Linda Cardozo**, Professor of Urogynaecology, Kings College Hospital, London – urogynaecology; **Dr Anna Glasier**, Consultant/Director of Family Planning & Well Women Services, Edinburgh – contraception; Professor Ian Greer, Muirhead Professor of Obstetrics and Gynaecology, Glasgow University, Glasgow – medical complications of pregnancy; **Dr Mary Hepburn**, Senior Lecturer in Obstetrics and Gynaecology, Glasgow University, Glasgow – drug misuse in pregnancy; **Dr Ian Lowles**, Consultant Obstetrician and Gynaecologist, Borders General Hospital, Melrose – gynaecological surgery; **Dr Lena Macara**, Consultant Obstetrician and Gynaecologist, Department of Fetal Medicine, Queen Mother's Hospital, Glasgow – pre-natal diagnosis and congenital abnormalities; **Dr Alan Mathers**, Consultant Obstetrician and Clinical Director, Glasgow Royal Maternity Hospital, Glasgow – acute obstetrics; **Dr David McKay Hart**, Consultant Gynaecologist, Stobhill Hospital, Glasgow – menopause; **Dr Philip Myerscough**, Consultant Obstetrician and Gynaecologist (Retd), Simpson Maternity Memorial Pavilion, Edinburgh – gynaecological surgery; **Dr Linda Myskow**, General Practitioner and Specialist in Sexual Health, Whinpark Medical Centre, Edinburgh – sexual health; **Dr Fiona Nelson**, Specialist Registrar in Obstetrics and Gynaecology with MPhil. in Medical Law and Ethics, South East Scotland Registrar Rotation – legal issues in obstetrics and gynaecology; **Dr Jane Norman**, Senior Lecturer in Obstetrics and Gynaecology, Glasgow University, Glasgow – general gynaecology; **Dr Philip Owen**, Consultant Obstetrician and Gynaecologist, Glasgow Royal Maternity Hospital, Glasgow – antenatal problems; **Dr Gordon Scott**, Consultant in Genitourinary Medicine, The Royal Infirmary of Edinburgh, Edinburgh – gynaecological infections; **Dr Nadeem Siddique**, Consultant Gynaecological Oncologist, Stobhill Hospital, Glasgow – gynaecological oncology; **Phil Toozs-Hobson**, Research Registrar, Kings College Hospital, London – urogynaecology.

I would also like to thank Miss Marion McKenzie, for endless letters and typing of 'must have it by this afternoon' paragraphs, and Mr Neil Bates of Siemens, for permission to reproduce selected ultrasound images.

I am most grateful to Dr Allan Gordon for his meticulous proof reading.

Abbreviations

αFP	α-fetoprotein	BCG	Bacille–Calmette–Guérin
ABGs	arterial blood gases	BD	bis die (twice a day)
AC	abdominal circumference	BM	Boehringer Mannheim
ACE	angiotensin converting enzyme	BMI	body mass index
		BP	blood pressure
ACTH	adrenocorticotrophic hormone	BPD	biparietal diameter
		BSO	bilateral salpingo-oophorectomy
AD	autosomal dominant		
AF	atrial fibrillation	BTS	blood transfusion service
AFI	amniotic fluid index		
AGA	appropriate for gestational age	CAH	congenital adrenal hyperplasia
AIDS	autoimmune deficiency syndrome	CCAM	congenital cystic adenomatoid malformation
AIN	anal intraepithelial neoplasia	CDH	congenital dislocated hip
AIS	adenocarcinoma in situ	CGMP	cyclic guanosine monophosphate
AITP	autoimmune thrombocytopenia purpura	CHB	congenital heart block
		CHD	congenital heart disease
ANF	antinuclear factor	CI	contraindicated
AP	anteroposterior	CIN	cervical intraepithelial neoplasia
APH	antepartum haemorrhage		
APTT	activated partial thromboplastin time	CMV	cytomegalovirus
		CNS	central nervous system
AR	autosomal recessive	COC	combined oral contraceptive
ARDS	adult respiratory distress syndrome		
		CP	cerebral palsy
ARF	acute renal failure	CPR	cardiopulmonary resuscitation
ARM	artificial rupture of membranes		
		CRP	c-reactive protein
ASAP	as soon as possible	CSF	cerebrospinal fluid
ASD	atrial septal defect	CT	computerized tomography
AST	aspartate transaminase	CTG	cardiotocograph
AV	atrioventricular	CVP	central venous pressure
AXR	abdominal X-ray	CVS	chorionic villus sampling
AZT	zidovudine	CXR	chest X-ray

DC	direct current	FSH	follicle stimulating
DHAS	dehydroepiandrosterone		hormone
	sulphate	FTA	fluorescent treponemal
DI	detrusor instability		antibody
DIC	disseminated		
	intravascular coagulation	G&S	group and save serum
DKA	diabetic ketoacidosis	G6PD	glucose-6-phosphatase
DUB	dysfunctional uterine		deficiency
	bleeding	GA	general anaesthetic
DVT	deep venous thrombosis	GFR	glomerular filtration rate
		GI	gastro-intestinal
ECG	electrocardiogram	GIFT	gamete intrafallopian
ECMO	extracorporeal membrane		transfer
	oxygenation	GnRH	gonadotrophin releasing
ECV	external cephalic version		hormone
ED	every day	GP	general practitioner
EDD	estimated date of	GSI	genuine stress
	delivery		incontinence
EDTA	ethylenediamine	GT	glucose tolerance
	tetraacetic acid	GTN	glyceryl trinitrate
EEG	electroencephalogram	GTT	glucose tolerance test
ELISA	enzyme linked	GU	genitourinary
	immunosorbent assay		
EMD	electromechanical	H'CRIT	haematocrit
	dissociation	Hb	haemoglobin
ERPOC	evacuation of retained	HBV	hepatitis B virus
	products of conception	hCG	human chorionic
ESR	erythrocyte		gonadotrophin
	sedimentation rate	HDL	high density lipoprotein
ET	endotracheal	HDN	haemolytic disease of the
EUA	examination under		newborn
	anaesthetic	HELLP	haemolysis, elevated liver
			enzymes, low platelets
FA	fetal anomaly	HIV	human
FBC	full blood count		immunodeficiency virus
FBS	fetal blood sample	hMG	human menopausal
FFP	fresh frozen plasma		gonadotrophin
FFTS	feto-fetal transfusion	HOCM	hypertrophic obstructive
	sequence		cardiomyopathy
FH	fetal heart	HPO	hypothalamopituitary–
FIGO	International Federation		ovarian
	of Gynaecologists and	HPV	human papilloma virus
	Obstetricians	HRT	hormone replacement
FL	femur length		therapy
FNA	fine-needle aspiration	HSG	hysterosalpingogram

HSV	herpes simplex virus	LFTs	liver function tests
HUS	haemolytic uraemic syndrome	LH	luteinizing hormone
HVS	high vaginal swab	LHRH	luteinizing hormone releasing hormone
IBD	inflammatory bowel disease	LLETZ	large loop electrodiathermy excision of the transformation zone
IBS	irritable bowel syndrome		
ICSI	intracytoplasmic sperm injection	LMP	last menstrual period
		LMW	low molecular weight
ICU	intensive care unit	LW	labour ward
IDDM	insulin dependent diabetes mellitus	MAOIs	monoamine oxidase inhibitors
Ig	immunoglobulin		
IHD	ischaemic heart disease	MAR	mixed antibody reaction
IM	intramuscular	MCH	mean corpuscular haemoglobin
INR	international normalized ratio	MCHC	mean corpuscular haemoglobin concentration
IOL	induction of labour		
IPPV	intermittent positive pressure ventilation	MCV	mean cell volume
		MF	multifactorial
ISSHP	International Society for the Study of Hypertension in Pregnancy	MI	myocardial infarction
		MMR	mumps, measles and rubella
		MMT	mixed Müllerian tumour
ISSVD	International Society for the Study of Vulval Diseases	MOM	multiples of the median
		MRC	Medical Research Council
ITU	intensive treatment unit	MRI	magnetic resonance imaging
IUCD	intra-uterine contraceptive device	MS	multiple sclerosis
IUD	intrauterine death	MSU	midstream urine
IUGR	intrauterine growth retardation	NGU	non-gonococcal urethritis
IV	intravenous	NIDDM	non-insulin-dependent diabetes mellitus
IVF	in vitro fertilization		
IVU	intravenous urogram	NS	not significant
		NSAIDs	non-steroidal anti-inflammatory drugs
KCT	kaolin clotting time		
		NT	nuchal translucency
LA	local anaesthetic	NTD	neural tube defect
LB	live birth	NYC	New York City
LCR	ligase chain reaction		
LDH	lactic dehydrogenase	OA	occipito-anterior
LDL	low density lipoprotein	OD	once daily

OD_{45}	optical density at 450 μm	RDS	respiratory distress syndrome
OP	occipitoposterior		
OT	occipitotransverse	RR	relative risk
		RUQ	right upper quadrant
P	pulse		
PA	pernicious anaemia	SANDS	Stillbirth and Neonatal Death Society
PCC	postcoital contraception		
PCOS	polycystic ovarian syndrome	SB	stillbirth
		SC	subcutaneously
PCR	polymerase chain	SCBU	special care baby unit
PDA	patent ductus arteriosis	SFD	small for dates
PG	prostaglandin	SGA	small for gestational age
PID	pelvic inflammatory disease	SHBG	sex hormone binding globulin
PMB	postmenopausal bleeding	SIDS	sudden infant death syndrome
PMS	premenstrual syndrome		
PN	postnatal	SLE	systemic lupus erythematosus
PO	per os (orally)		
POG	Progress in Obstetrics and Gynaecology	SRM	spontaneous rupture of the membranes
POP	progestogen-only pill	SSRI	selective serotonin reuptake inhibitor
PPH	postpartum haemorrhage		
PPROM	preterm prelabour rupture of the membranes	stat	statim (at once)
		STD	sexually transmitted disease
PPV	positive predictive value		
Prl	prolactin	SVD	spontaneous vertex delivery
PROM	prelabour rupture of the membranes		
		SVT	supraventricular tachycardia
PTE	pulmonary thromboembolus		
PTR	prothrombin ratio	T13	trisomy 13
PUVA	ultraviolet A with psoralen	T18	trisomy 18
		T21	trisomy 21
PV	per vaginam	T_4	thyroxine
		TA	transabdominal
QID	quarter in die (four times a day)	TAH	total abdominal hysterectomy
		TB	tuberculosis
RAFEA	radio frequency endometrial ablation	3TC	lamivudine
		TCRE	transcervical resection of endometrium
RBBB	right bundle branch block		
RCC	red cell concentrate	TFT	thyroid function test
RCOG	Royal College of Obstetricians and Gynaecologists	TIA	transient ischaemic attack
		TID	ter in die (three times a day)

TOP	termination of pregnancy		VDRL	venereal diseases reference laboratories
TORCH	toxoplasmosis, rubella, CMV, HSV		VE	vaginal examination
TPHA	*Treponema pallidum* haemagglutination		VF	ventricular fibrillation
			VIN	vulval intraepithelial neoplasia
TPN	total parenteral nutrition		VQ	ventilation–perfusion
TSH	thyroid stimulating hormone		VSD	ventricular septal defect
TV	transvaginal		VT	ventricular tachycardia
TZ	transitional zone		VUR	vesicoureteric reflux
			VZIG	varicella zoster immunoglobulin
U&E	urea and electrolytes			
uE3	unconjugated oestriol			
USS	ultrasound scan		WCC	white cell count
UTI	urinary tract infection		WHO	World Health Organization
VACTERL	vertebral, anal, cardiac, tracheal, oesophageal, renal and limb		XL	X-linked
VAIN	vaginal intraepithelial neoplasia		ZIFT	zygote intrafallopian transfer
VATER	vertebral, anal, tracheal, oesophageal and renal		ZIG	zoster immunoglobulin

CHAPTER I

PRENATAL DIAGNOSIS AND CONGENITAL ABNORMALITIES

INTRODUCTION

Ideally, if the parents of a baby with a congenital anomaly can be seen by the same person at each clinic visit, it may go a long way towards easing anxiety. If a serious problem develops and there is a lot of parental anxiety, do not be afraid to allow parents to contact you personally at the hospital – most do not and the point of contact will be a reassurance.

The finding of some 'abnormality' in pregnancy transforms what was previously an exciting and joyous event into an extremely worrying and distressing time. This remains true even when the potential risks are small; for example being recalled with an abnormal αFP, or with the finding of a choroid plexus cyst on routine ultrasound scan. The very greatest of care should be taken in explaining any findings to parents. Tact, understanding and reassurance (if appropriate) are paramount. The advice we give parents is of such importance that it will frequently be necessary to involve senior members of the obstetrics team as well as members of other specialties, particularly paediatricians, clinical geneticists and radiologists. The details provided here are simplified versions of what are frequently complex diagnostic problems with very uncertain outcomes, and possession of this book is not an excuse to deny parents access to specialists in this field.

Aims of prenatal diagnosis

These aims are fourfold:

- the identification at an early gestation of abnormalities incompatible with survival, or likely to result in severe handicap, in order to prepare parents and offer the option of termination of pregnancy;
- the identification of conditions which may influence the timing, site or mode of delivery;
- the identification of fetuses who would benefit from early paediatric intervention;
- the identification of fetuses who may benefit from in utero treatment (rare).

The first aim is usually the most controversial. Do not assume that all parents are going to request TOP even in the presence of lethal abnormality. Many couples have opted to continue pregnancies in the face of severe defects which have resulted in either intrauterine or early neonatal death, and have expressed the view that they found it easier to cope with grief having held their child. Others say that they were glad of the opportunity to terminate the pregnancy at an early stage and that they could not have coped with going on. More controversial still are the problems of chronic diseases with long-term handicap and long-term suffering for both the child and its parents. The parents themselves must decide what action they wish to take – it is they who will have to live with the decisions we place in front of them. It is our role to advise, guide and respect their final wishes, irrespective of our own personal views.

As thalamocortical connections do not develop until >22 weeks, it is not possible for the fetus to feel pain before this gestation. Analgesia may be used for procedures >24 weeks, but it is unlikely that there is fetal 'awareness' until 26 weeks.

NORMAL VIEWS FOR BPD, AC AND FL

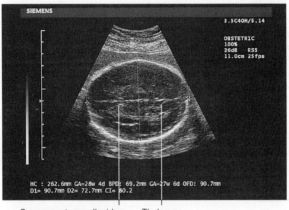

Cavum septum pellucidum   Thalamus

Fig. 1.1 Normal biparietal diameter. (Reproduced with permission from Siemens.)

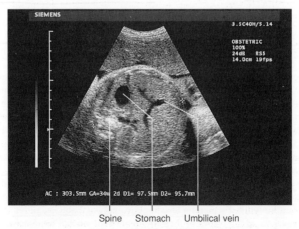

Spine   Stomach   Umbilical vein

Fig. 1.2 Normal abdominal circumference. (Reproduced with permission from Siemens.)

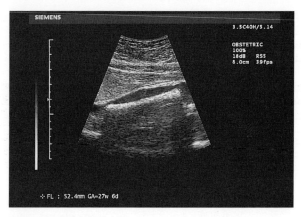

Fig. 1.3 Normal femur length. (Reproduced with permission from Siemens.)

SCREENING FOR FETAL ABNORMALITIES

Structural anomalies are best seen on ultrasound scan, and many clinicians advocate that all mothers should be offered at least one detailed ultrasound at around 18–20 weeks or earlier. This has the advantage that previously unsuspected major or lethal anomalies (e.g. spina bifida, renal agenesis) can be offered termination, and it also allows planned deliveries when conditions are present which may require early neonatal intervention (e.g. gastroschisis, transposition of the great arteries). It has the disadvantage, however, that many defects are not identified (it is likely that <50% of cardiac defects are recognized) and the false reassurance provided by this scan may become a source of parental resentment. Furthermore, some problem may be uncovered, for example one of the 'soft markers' (see below), the natural history of which is uncertain. This may generate unnecessary anxiety and increase the number of invasive diagnostic procedures (and thereby the loss rate) in otherwise healthy pregnancies. The results of studies into the benefits of routine scanning have been conflicting (N Engl J Med 1993:821, Br Med J 1993:13) and depend to a large degree on the skill of the sonographer.

Chromosomal abnormalities are much more difficult to identify on scan. While around two-thirds of fetuses with Down's syndrome will look normal at 18 weeks, most Edward's and Patau's syndromes do show some abnormality, even though these are often not specific or diagnostic. The two most commonly used screening tests for chromosomal abnormalities are serum markers at ≥15 weeks or measurement of the nuchal translucency at 11–14 weeks.

SERUM SCREENING

Antental screening for Down's syndrome is possible by examining levels of serum markers at ≥15 weeks' gestation, particularly low levels of αFP ±high levels of unconjugated oestriol and hCG. By correcting these for maternal weight and adjusting the results for maternal age, ≈60% of cases of Down's syndrome can be picked up by carrying out amniocentesis on ≈4% of the screened population (N Engl J Med 1992:588). The cut-off for recall is usually >1:250. The pick-up rate is higher in older women, but the chance of being recalled with an elevated risk is also higher (Table 1.1). It is therefore not essential to advise women over the age of 35 years to have an amniocentesis, as serum screening is more sensitive in this age group.

TABLE 1.1   Serum screening for Down's syndrome according to age of mother

Age of mother (years)	Sensitivity (%) (ie number of cases picked up)	Recalled (%)
<25	35	2
25–29	40	3
30–34	54	7
35		13
36		19
37	76	19
38		26
39		32
40–44	93	44
>45	>99	85

Amniocentesis carries a miscarriage rate of 0.5–1%. In addition, 0.5–1% will fail to culture and 0.25–1% will show mosaicism confirmed in only 50% of fetuses. Amniocentesis before 15 weeks carries a greater chance of miscarriage. Karyotype results are usually available within 3 weeks, but FISH (fluorescence in situ hybridization) techniques may be used to exclude the commoner aneuploidies within 72 hours. (see Table 1.2.)

TABLE 1.2 Association between maternal serum markers and specified fetal abnormalities

	T21	T18	T13	XO	Triploid	Hydrops	IUD
αFP	↓	↓↓	Usually normal	Usually normal	? ↑	↓	↑	↑
hCG	↑	↓↓	Usually normal	Slight ↓*	? ↓	↓	↓	↑
uE₃	↑	↓↓	Usually normal		? ↓ or normal	↑	↓	
	60% sensitivity for 4% false positive	50–60% sensitivity for 0.3% false positive.	Unless NTD	*hCG may be slight ↑ with hydrops		↑ αFP even demise	Poor prognosis	

Screening for open neural tube defects is also carried out by measuring the maternal serum αFP at 16 weeks (see also p. 14). It is generally accepted that those with levels greater than 2.0–2.5 multiples of the median should be recalled for an ultrasound scan, giving a sensitivity of around 85%. Maternal serum αFP may also be elevated following first-trimester bleeding, or with intrauterine death, twins, abdominal wall defects, congenital nephrosis, Turner syndrome, epidermolysis bullosa, rhesus disease and renal agenesis. It is important to bear in mind that, even if the ultrasound scan is normal, an elevated αFP is still a marker for later pre-eclampsia or IUGR (Table 1.3) (Prenat Diag 1995;15(11):1041). There is evidence that Doppler studies may help to differentiate this group (Br J Obstet Gynaecol 1998; (suppl 17): abstract 198). If the αFP and hCG are raised, at least 60% are likely to have some complication (Am J Perinatol 1995;12(2):93).

TABLE 1.3 Associations following raised αFP and normal ultrasound scan

	Extremely SGA (< 2.2nd centile)	SGA (< 10th centile)	Preterm delivery (AGA)
↑ αFP (> 2.5 MOM)	9.4% (RR 4.5)	27% (RR 2.7)	14% (RR 2.4)
↑ hCG	4.4% (RR 2.1)	15% (RR 1.5)	NS
↑ αFP + hCG	24% (RR 10.9)	38%	47% (RR 3.0)

NUCHAL TRANSLUCENCY

Screening is also possible by measuring the fetal nuchal thickness on first trimester ultrasound between 11–14 weeks (Fig. 1.4). Sensitivities of around 70–80% (higher by adding serum markers) have been quoted for detecting Down's syndrome; (N Engl J Med 1998;955 and Lancet 1998;352:343). The sensitivity of NT screening may appear artificially higher than serum screening because of spontaneous losses between 12 and 16 weeks. CVS may be used to establish an earlier diagnosis (≥11 weeks), allowing a surgical termination of pregnancy. There is, however, good evidence to suggest that psychological parental morbidity is independent of whether a diagnosis is made in the first or second trimester, and indeed medical TOP may carry less psychological morbidity than surgical TOP (even if medical complications are higher). In very experienced hands, CVS at 11–14 weeks may carry the same complication rate as amniocentesis at 16 weeks, but for most practitioners CVS probably carries a higher risk of miscarriage (2–3%). One per cent will show mosaicism which is limited to the placenta and does not affect the fetus (confined placental mosaicism), but errors from this can be virtually eliminated if decisions are deferred until both the direct and culture results are available. Karyotypic discrepancy between fetus and placenta increases with increasing gestation and if rapid results are required >20 weeks, FBS or amniocentesis with fluorescence in situ hybridization (FISH) is preferable.

Increased NT is also a marker for structural defects (4% of those >3 mm), particularly cardiac, diaphragmatic hernia, renal, abdominal wall and other more rare abnormalities (US Obstet Gynecol 1998;11:391). The overall survival for those with NT >5 mm is ≈53%.

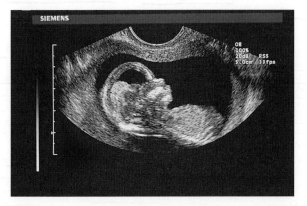

Fig. 1.4 Saggital view for nuchal translucency measurement. (Reproduced with permission from Siemens.)

ANEUPLOIDY

SYNDROMES

TRISOMY 21 (Down's syndrome) (see also Screening, p. 4)

The overall incidence is 1:650 LBs, but the individual incidence is dependent on maternal age. Most Down's syndrome children, however, are born to younger mothers as they have proportionately more babies. Although walking, language and self-care skills are usually attained, independence is rare. There is mental retardation (with a mean IQ around 50) and an association with CHD (particularly AV canal defects, VSD, PDA, ASD primum and Fallot's tetralogy). GI atresias are common, and there is early dementia with similarities to Alzheimer's disease. Twenty per cent die before the age of 1 year and 45% reach 60 years old.

Incidence

The incidence increases with advancing maternal age:

20 years	1:2000	38 years	1:180
30 years	1:900	40 years	1:100
35 years	1:350	44 years	1:40
36 years	1:240		

handwritten notes:
- Duod. atresia
- Diaph. hernia
- prolonged parental support
- Special school
- Ac leukemia

Overall, 95% of cases are due to non-dysjunction, with translocation 14:21 accounting for 2%, other translocations 2% and mosaicism 1%. Half of the translocations occur de novo. The recurrence risk for non-dysjunction is an additional 0.75% above the background risk. If there is a 14:21 translocation in the mother the recurrence risk is 1:10, and 1:50 if this translocation is present in the father.

Trisomy 18 (Edward's syndrome)

Incidence 1:2500 LBs. Most are due to non-dysjunction. The baby has IUGR, a small elongated head (strawberry shaped on USS), severe mental retardation, rocker bottom feet and an increased incidence of GI and renal anomalies. CHD is almost invariable (usually VSD, ASD or PDA), and overlapping fingers and flexion deformities may also be seen. Overall, 50% die before the age of 2 months and 90% before the end of the first year.

Trisomy 13 (Patau's syndrome)

Incidence 1:5000 LBs. Overall, 75% of cases are due to non-dysjunction. There is IUGR, severe mental retardation and an increased incidence of cleft palate, GI atresias and holoprosencephaly. In 80% of cases there is CHD. The majority of children die before the age of 3 months, and rarely survive after the age of 1 year. A very small number may survive for years.

Triploidy

Fetuses rarely survive to birth and there is no survival beyond the neonatal period.

XO (Turner's syndrome)

Incidence 1:3000 LBs. Overall, 60% of cases are pure XO, ≥15% are mosaics (usually XO/XX) and the rest are deletions, rings or isochromosomes of Xq or Xp. The incidence is increased with increasing paternal age and decreased with increasing maternal age. Antenatally there may be a cystic hygroma ± generalized oedema and cardiac defects. Postnatally there may be short stature, cubitus valgus, coarctation of the aorta, a bicuspid aortic valve, streak gonads and, only occasionally, a lowered IQ. A small proportion may be fertile (particularly mosaics and deletions), although the incidence of premature ovarian failure is greater. The risks of pregnancy loss and karyotypic abnormalities in the fetus are also greater.

XXX

1:1000 LBs. The incidence is doubled or tripled when the maternal age is more than 40 years. The phenotype and fertility are normal and the abnormality frequently goes unnoticed. There is, however, an increased risk of sex chromosome abnormalities (≈4%) and premature menopause in the offspring.

XXX + (ie more than three X chromosomes)

This is rare. Dysmorphism and mental retardation are common, as is menstrual dysfunction. The individual may be fertile.

XXY (Klinefelter's syndrome)

1:700–2000 LBs. The incidence is increased with advanced maternal age. The individual is phenotypically a tall male, with an occasionally reduced IQ, sparse facial hair and gynaecomastia. It is the commonest single cause of male hypogonadism and is usually diagnosed in the investigation of male infertility. There is an association with hypothyroidism, diabetes and asthma. Azoospermia is the rule.

XYY

1:700 LBs. The incidence of this is not associated with maternal age. The IQ and fertility are usually normal and the suggestion of increased impulsive behaviour may be biased by the population sampled. Individuals are usually tall. The risk of sex chromosome abnormalities in offspring is ≈4%.

Apparently balanced rearrangements (translocations or inversions)

If found at amniocentesis it is essential to karyotype the parents. If one parent has the translocation and is phenotypically normal, it is likely that the fetus will be phenotypically normal as well. There is a chance that other offspring (or offspring of the fetus) will have an unbalanced translocation and counselling ± karyotyping should be offered. In general the smaller the section of chromosome involved, the greater the likelihood of a fetus surviving to term with an unbalanced translocation. Offspring may, of course, also have normal karyotypes without the translocation. If the translocation has occurred de novo, the overall risk of phenotypic abnormality is in the order of 10% but as some chromosomal re-arrangements are normal population variants, genetic advice should always be sought.

Unbalanced chromosomal structural abnormalities

Many abnormalities are well characterised, but it is often difficult to be specific. Parental karyotyping is required and genetic advice should be sought. Mental impairment is common, and physical abnormality is possible.

SOFT MARKERS

These are structural features found on USS which in themselves are not a problem, but which may be pointers to aneuploidy. They are found in ≈5% of all pregnancies in the second trimester and are the cause of a lot of parental anxiety. Assignment of risk for aneuploidy is fraught with difficulty as adequate data from low-risk pregnancies are very limited. If isolated, the risk of chromosomal problems is low (see below). If more than one soft marker is found, or if there are any other structural defects, the risk is very much higher (RCOG Review 97/09). The more subtle markers (clinodactyly, sandal gap, polydactyly, etc.) are not discussed here.

Borderline ventriculomegaly

The normal ventricle measures 6.6 ± 1.2 mm; 10 mm is >3 SD. Ventriculomegaly is said to be present if one or both of the ventricles measures >10 mm. The risk of aneuploidy is ≈ × 1.5 the baseline risk. → 5 - 10%

Choroid plexus cysts

The choroid plexus may demonstrate small cysts *with hyperechoic capsules* (up to about 10 mm in diameter) in early pregnancy. These are present in 1% of all 18-week scans, are often bilateral, are thought to be developmental in origin and usually disappear by 24 weeks' gestation. There is an association with T18 and T13, although probably no association with T21. If other abnormalities are present the risk of aneuploidy is high. If isolated, maternal age should be considered before the decision to karyotype is taken (Br J Obstet Gynaecol 1997;104:881), e.g. the risk of T18 at 20 years is 1:500, at 30 years is 1:300 and at 40 years is 1:37. Both resolution and size are unrelated to karyotype risk.

Echogenic bowel

Echogenic bowel is a midtrimester finding which occurs in less than 1% of pregnancies. The bowel is bright, being similar to the spine/ribs in echogenicity. There is an association with aneuploidy (≈3%), cystic fibrosis ~~TORCH~~ (0–13%) and perinatal death (≈10%). Parents should be tested for cystic ~~geihia~~ fibrosis mutations and fetal karyotyping should be considered (see p. 28). A normal outcome can be anticipated in about two-thirds of cases overall, and in 84% in whom hyperechogenic bowel is an isolated finding.

Echogenic foci

There is a moving echogenic focus (or 'golf ball') within either or both cardiac ventricles which has no obvious anatomically associated structure, but may represent papillary microcalcification (Fig. 1.5). The incidence is ≈3%. Structural heart disease should be excluded (see p. 12). There may be a slightly increased risk of T21, but this risk is probably less than 1% with isolated lesions (Obstet Gynecol 1997;89:945).

Renal pelvic dilatation

This is defined as a dilatation of >4mm before 33 weeks and >7mm after 33 weeks (Fig. 1.6). The T21 and T18 risk is increased approximately 1.5-fold over age-related risk alone. If serum or NT screening for aneuploidy has already been carried out, however, almost certainly no further action is required (Br J Obstet Gynaecol 1998:860). There is also an association with postnatal reflux, UTI and renal scarring (see p. 21).

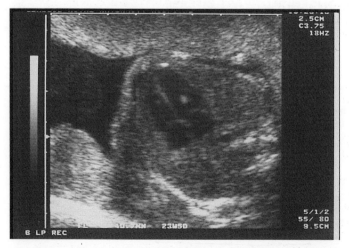

Fig. 1.5 Left ventricular echogenic focus in an otherwise normal four-chamber view at 20 weeks' gestation. There was a normal outcome.

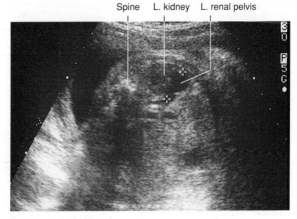

Fig. 1.6 Left renal pelvic dilatation at 33 weeks gestation. This resolved postnatally.

Nuchal translucency
See page 7.

See page 7.

STRUCTURAL DISORDERS

CONGENITAL HEART DISEASE

> This is the commonest congenital malformation in children and affects about 5–8:1000 live births. Approximately 2–3 of these 8 are severe malformations. Of defects diagnosed antenatally, about 15% are associated with aneuploidy, most commonly T18 and T21.

Antenatal diagnosis
Certain groups carry a greater risk of CHD particularly in those:

- with extracardiac anomalies (20%),
- with a CHD in either parent (particularly the mother) or a sibling (2–6%) (Lancet 1998;351:311),
- with diabetes mellitus (3%, although possibly less with better diabetic control in the first trimester),
- who have been exposed to teratogens, particularly lithium and anticonvulsants,
- with fetal arrhythmias, particularly CHB (P < 100 bpm),
- with non-immune hydrops fetalis,
- with increased NT between 10 and 14 weeks.

The four-chamber view of the heart can be used as a screening test and will identify 25–40% of all major abnormalities (see Fig. 1.5). In addition, viewing the aorta and pulmonary artery increases the sensitivity to ≥60%. At 18 weeks most of the major connections can be seen, but high-risk pregnancies should be rescanned at 22–26 weeks to identify more minor defects. When a problem is identified, the patient should be referred to a tertiary scanning centre for a more detailed structural assessment and Doppler studies.

Scanning fetal hearts

Check that the heart is on the left and obtain a four-chamber view. Deviation of the cardiac axis to the left (>75° from midline) and the right (<25°) is strongly associated with structural abnormality. The heart should occupy approximately one-third of the thorax and have a normal, regular rhythm (use M-mode if necessary). Look at contractility and check for pericardial effusion. The right ventricle lies behind the sternum, and the left atrium (with its connecting pulmonary veins) is in front of the descending thoracic aorta. Both ventricles should be the same size (one small ventricle suggests left- or right-sided hypoplasia), and the interventricular septum, when viewed at 90° to the direction of scanning, should be intact (i.e. no VSDs). The right ventricle has a moderator band at its apex and the tricuspid valve is inserted a little more towards the apex than the mitral valve. While the valves should close synchronously, they should be seen to move independently.

By inclining the transducer more cephalad, it is possible to see the aortic outflow from the left ventricle in the direction of the right fetal shoulder and, further cephalad, the pulmonary artery. This arises from the right ventricle and crosses the aorta at approximately 90° on its way posteriorly (a pulmonary artery parallel to the aorta suggests transposition of the great arteries). The anterior wall of the aorta should be continuous with the interventricular septum (discontinuity suggests VSD or endocardial cushion defect) and should not override the interventricular septum (suggests Fallot's tetralogy).

Arrhythmias

You should involve fetal medicine specialists.

Irregular. Usually premature atrial contractions (extrasystolic beats, dropped beats). Ventricular ectopic beats are very rare. Only 1–2% proceed to a tachyarrhythmia, and the risk of structural heart disease is only 1–2%.

Bradycardia. Usually congenital heart block (atrial movement appears independent of the ventricle). Exclude maternal SLE (see p. 111). If there is abnormal anatomy, the prognosis is very poor. If structurally normal, the prognosis is variable:

- if hydropic, <50% survive;
- if not, almost always OK;
- if FH rate decreases or is <50 bpm the prognosis is less good.

Postnatal pacing may be required. In utero treatment by maternal administration of steroids has occasionally been associated with resolution; the benefit of chronotropic agents is very uncertain.

Tachyarrhythmias. Almost always SVT with a rate of 220–240 bpm. Atrial flutter/fibrillation is less common and ventricular tachycardia is only rarely reported. The presence of hydrops is associated with a poorer prognosis. Diagnosis and management should be coordinated in a tertiary referral unit. Treatment options are limited. Both digoxin and flecainide have both been used successfully, but are potentially toxic to the mother.

CRANIOSPINAL DEFECTS (MF)

Neural tube defects (see also Screening, p. 5)

- *Anencephaly*: the skull vault and cerebral cortex are absent.
- *Spina bifida*:
  — meningocele: dura and arachnoid mater bulge through the defect;
  — myelomeningocele: the central canal of the cord is exposed.
- *Encephalocele*: there is a bony defect in the cranial vault through which a dura mater sac (±brain tissue) protrudes.

Spina bifida and anencephaly make up more than 95% of NTDs. There is wide geographical variation in births, with a higher incidence in Scotland and Ireland (3:1000), and a lower incidence in England (2:1000), the USA, Canada, Japan and Africa (<1:1000). There is good evidence that the overall incidence has fallen over the past 15 years (independent of any screening programmes).

Recurrence risk is:

- with 1 affected sibling,   1:25;
- with 2 or more affected siblings, 1:10;
- with 1 affected parent,   1:25.

Anencephaly The infant is either stillborn or, if liveborn, will usually die shortly after birth (although some may survive for several days).

Spina bifida The spine can be viewed by ultrasound in three planes to assess the type and level of any deficit (Fig. 1.7). Hydrocephalus occurs in about 90% of fetuses with spina bifida and carries a much poorer prognosis than spina bifida alone. Markers for spina bifida (which are 99% sensitive) include blunting of the sinciput (the lemon sign, Fig. 1.8), a banana-shaped cerebellum (Arnold–Chiari malformation) and an absent cerebellum (Fig. 1.9). Those with myelomeningoceles usually have abnormal lower limb neurology, and many have hydrocephalus. In addition to immobility and mental retardation there may be problems with UTI, bladder dysfunction, bowel dysfunction, and social and sexual isolation. 90% are handicapped and 30% live to 5 years of age.

Encephalocele This may be occipital or frontal. Isolated meningoceles carry a good prognosis, whereas those with microcephaly secondary to brain herniation carry a very poor prognosis. As more than 95% of encephaloceles are closed defects, the maternal serum αFP level is usually normal.

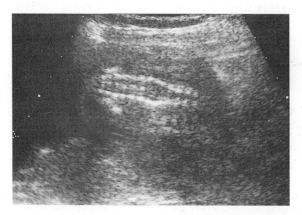

Fig. 1.7 Coronal view of spina bifida with dysraphism of the thoracolumbar vertebral bodies.

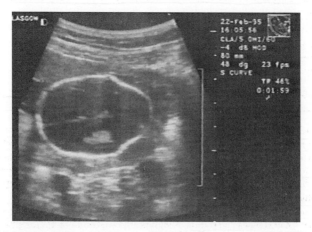

Fig. 1.8 Lemon-shaped skull of a fetus with spina bifida.

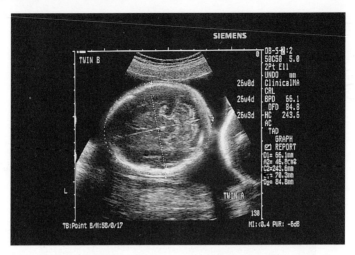

Fig. 1.9 A normal cerebellum. Spina bifida is very unlikely. (Reproduced with permission from Siemens.)

Prevention

The MRC Vitamin Study Group (1991) showed that folate 4 mg/day PO taken from before conception reduced the recurrence risk of NTDs in those who had had an affected child previously. A preconceptual prophylactic dose of 400 µg/day PO for all pregnant women may be more physiological, and use of this dose is supported by earlier studies. There are, at present, no known teratogenic effects of folate.

Microcephaly

Most microcephalies are MF, but a few are AR. The head circumference is three standard deviations below the expected value compared to the rest of the measurements (e.g. abdominal circumference, femur length). The children are frequently mentally retarded, often severely. In general, the smaller the head the worse the prognosis, but children have developed normally despite very small head circumferences. The condition may occur following infection (particularly rubella), as part of a multiple malformation syndrome, or secondary to some other teratogen, but in most cases the cause is never established. In the absence of a known cause, the recurrence risk is 1:10. The diagnosis requires serial ultrasound scanning and is frequently not made until at least 24 weeks' gestation. A significant proportion of microcephalies are missed prenatally.

Ventriculomegaly

[handwritten annotations: 5–10% chr. ab^t / 50% die by 1yr / 50% serious neurological sequelae.]

Ventriculomegaly may be taken as a lateral ventricular atrium measurement of >10 mm (Fig. 1.10). The head is usually normal sized. Hydrocephaly may be taken as further dilatation with thinning and 'dangling' of the dependent choroid plexus, and head size may (but does not necessarily) increase above centiles in later pregnancy.

Ventriculomegaly has a 30% association with spina bifida (see above). Those cases not associated with spina bifida may occur secondary to obstruction, usually at the aqueduct of Sylvius (with a normal 4th ventricle) or at the foraminae of Luschka and Magendi (the Dandy–Walker malformation); the latter carries a poor prognosis (note that there are variants of this condition). Rare forms of ventriculomegaly include holoprosencephaly (absent cavum septum pellucidum and a single cerebral ventricle – associated with T13) and agenesis of the corpus callosum (absent cavum septum pellucidum, 3rd ventricle dilatation and separation of the anterior horns of the lateral ventricles), both of which carry a very poor prognosis. There is also an association with chromosomal disorders, particularly if severe and in the presence of other abnormalities, although idiopathic borderline ventriculomegaly (10–12 mm) carries only a small risk of aneuploidy (p. 10).

The prognosis of isolated ventriculomegaly is generally good unless the condition is progressive or severe. The prognosis is generally poor when other abnormalities are present. The recurrence risk for isolated hydrocephalus is about 1:30, but the much rarer sex-linked aqueduct stenosis carries a 1:4 risk of recurrence (1:2 if the fetus is already known to be male).

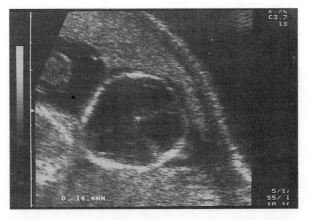

Fig. 1.10 Hydrocephalus. Note the dangling choroid plexus in the lower dilated ventricle.

GASTROINTESTINAL DISORDERS

Abdominal wall defects   *1/6000 incidence*

These may present because of an elevated serum maternal αFP.

Umb. cord is midline

Exomphalos (Fig. 1.11) This occurs following failure of the gut to return to the abdominal cavity at 8 weeks' gestation and results in a defect through which the peritoneal sac protrudes. This may contain both intestines and liver. There are chromosomal abnormalities in 30% (especially T18), and 10–50% have other lesions, particularly cardiac and renal. There is also an association with ectopia vesiciae and ectopia cardia. If the exomphalos is isolated (i.e. there are no other structural abnormalities), the chromosomes are normal and there is no bowel atresia or infarction, the prognosis is good (>80% long-term survival). The sac rarely ruptures at vaginal delivery. There is an association with Beckwith–Wiedmann syndrome (see p. 28). *Umb cord is attached to the apex of the sac.*

Gastroschisis (Fig. 1.12) This is commoner than exomphalos. The abdominal wall defect is usually to the right and below the insertion of the umbilical cord. Small bowel (without a peritoneal covering) protrudes and floats free in the peritoneal fluid. Gut atresias and cardiac lesions occur in 20% of cases, but the association with chromosomal abnormality is very small (probably <1%). The prognosis is good if the bowel is viable, although 10% of cases end in stillbirth despite apparently normal growth. Gut dilatation may be associated with bowel obstruction or ischaemia, but is not directly linked to prognosis. These babies are usually SFD and require very close surveillance. The recurrence risk is <1%.

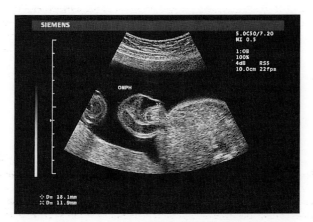

Fig. 1.11 A small exomphalos. (Reproduced with permission from Siemens.)

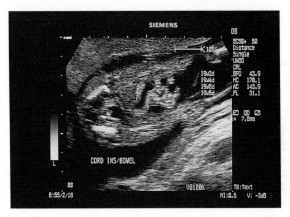

Fig. 1.12 Gastroschisis. (Reproduced with permission from Siemens.)

Bowel obstruction (MF)

Incidence 1:12 000 LBs. These are probably secondary to a vascular insult in early fetal life. There are multiple distended loops of bowel. The prognosis depends on the site of obstruction, the more distal carrying the better prognosis.

Duodenal atresia (MF)

Incidence 1:7000 LBs. The stomach and proximal duodenum distend to give the classic ultrasound double-bubble appearance and there is polyhydramnios. This may not be apparent on the 18 week scan, but is usually present by 25 weeks. There are other congenital malformations in 50%, including bowel, kidney and skeletal abnormalities. In 30% of cases there is T21. Jejunal atresia produces a triple-bubble appearance.

Echogenic bowel

See page 11.

Oesophageal atresia (MF)

Incidence 1:3000 LBs. The oesophagus is not readily seen on ultrasound, but the absence of a stomach bubble in the presence of polyhydramnios should raise the possibility of this diagnosis. In 90% of cases, however, there is a tracheo-oesophageal fistula which allows stomach filling, and the classic signs mentioned above are only present in one-third of cases. There is an association with aneuploidy in 15%, and also with cardiac defects.

GENITOURINARY ABNORMALITIES

Cystic disease

Isolated cysts arising from the substance of the kidney are rare, and only become significant if they are so large that they prevent a vaginal delivery. It may not be possible to establish a precise diagnosis antenatally.

Renal dysplasia

Multicystic dysplastic kidneys (sporadic inheritance) The kidneys have large discrete non-communicating cysts with a central, more solid core and are thought to follow early developmental failure (Fig. 1.13). If the cysts affect only one kidney, the other is normal, and there is adequate liquor, the prognosis is good. If the cysts are bilateral and the liquor is reduced, the prognosis is poor.

Dysplasia associated with congenital urinary tract obstruction This may occur if obstruction is severe and typically presents with small cortical cysts.

Polycystic kidney disease

Adult polycystic kidney disease (AD) The corticomedullary junction is accentuated and the condition is relatively benign, often not producing symptoms until the fifth decade of life. Many individuals have ultrasonically normal kidneys at birth. There are at least two genes on different chromosomes, however, so that DNA studies are only possible in families with multiple affected members.

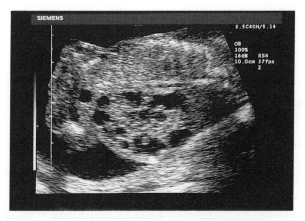

Fig. 1.13 Large multicystic dysplastic kidney. (Reproduced with permission from Siemens.)

Infantile polycystic kidney disease (AR) There is a wide range of expression, with the size of cysts ranging from microscopic to several millimetres across. Both kidneys are affected, and there may also be cysts present in the liver and pancreas. Ultrasound features of oligohydramnios, empty bladder and large symmetrical bright kidneys (Fig. 1.14) may not develop until later in pregnancy. Check for occipital encephalocele. If there is survival beyond the neonatal period, there may be later problems with raised BP and progressive renal failure. Long-term survival is rare.

Obstruction

Urinary tract obstruction occurs at three main sites, as described below.

Pyelectasis (see also p. 11 and Fig. 1.6) This may be unilateral (79–90%) or bilateral. It is probably caused by a neuromuscular defect at the junction of the ureter and the renal pelvis, which presents with increasing pelvic dilatation in the presence of a normal ureter. The cortical thickness is usually well preserved, but the kidney should be scanned repeatedly to monitor the cortical thickness (increased echogenicity and hydroureter carry a poorer prognosis). There is rarely any indication for induction of labour. As there is an association with postnatal UTIs and reflux nephropathy, it is reasonable to start all neonates on prophylactic antibiotics and arrange postnatal radiological follow-up (e.g. USS at 1–4 weeks, depending on severity, ± later micturating cystourethrogram). Even in those with mild dilatation (≥5 and <10 mm) there is VUR in 10–20%, although only a small proportion require surgery (US Obstet Gynecol 1997:12).

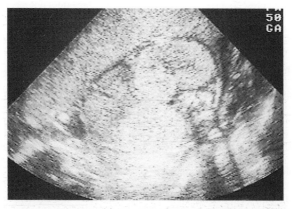

Fig. 1.14 Infantile polycystic kidney disease with anhydramnios at 26 weeks. The outcome was spontaneous intrauterine demise 2 weeks later.

Posterior urethral valves Folds of mucosa at the bladder neck prevent urine leaving the bladder. The fetus is usually male, there is often oligohydramnios, and on ultrasound there are varying degrees of renal dysplasia. There is a chromosomal abnormality in 7% of isolated defects and in one-third of those with other abnormalities. If the chromosomes are normal, the obstruction is severe and urinary electrolytes are normal, it is possible to insert a pigtail shunt between the bladder and amniotic cavity. This may relieve the obstruction, but the long-term prognosis is still poor as the renal damage may not be reversible.

Urethral stenosis There is usually marked oligohydramnios with dilatation of the urinary bladder, often with bilateral dysplastic kidneys. The outcome is usually fetal demise, but single bladder puncture or pigtail catheter insertion have been used.

Potter syndrome (MF – sporadic)

Incidence 1:10 000 LBs. Bilateral renal agenesis is associated with extreme oligohydramnios and leads to the Potter's sequence of pulmonary hypoplasia (see p. 24) and limb deformity. The condition is lethal (and indeed severe midtrimester oligohydramnios from any cause carries a relatively poor prognosis) (US Obstet Gynecol 1996:108). Fetal ultrasound diagnosis is problematic because the low liquor level makes visualization difficult; transvaginal scanning and fluid installation are of help. There may be associated cardiac abnormalities. Adrenal glands can be mistaken for kidneys (in the absence of kidneys, the adrenals expand to fill the space). Serial scanning over a few hours to look for bladder filling is important (evidence of no renal function). This also helps to avoid confusion with ectopic kidneys. Renal arteries (as seen with Doppler) are only present if kidneys are present (although the presence of a kidney does not mean that it is functioning). The recurrence risk is approximately 3%, although AD forms with variable penetrance have been described.

HAEMOGLOBIN VARIANTS AND THALASSAEMIA

Haemoglobin is composed of four subunits, each made up of a globin chain and a haem component. Normal adult haemoglobin is made up of 2α- and 2β-globin chains. Disorders affecting the structure or synthesis of these chains are known as haemoglobinopathies. Screening may be targeted, based on ethnic background, but caucasians may occasionally be carriers.

Disorders of globin structure

Haemoglobin structural variants result from a genetically determined chemical alteration in the globin molecule. There are many different pathological types, of which sickle-cell disease, a β-chain variant due to a single constant mutation, is the commonest.

Sickle-cell disease (AR)

This presents after the age of 6 months and, although 25% die before the age of 5 years, 50% survive to the age of 40. 'Crises', which may be precipitated by infection, dehydration, cold, hypoxia and stasis, affect joints, the back, long bones and spleen. In pregnancy there is an increased risk of pulmonary embolism and renal infarction. There is also a high fetal loss rate and increased chance of IUGR and prematurity. Maintain hydration, treat infection aggressively and transfuse only if the Hb much lower than usual for that patient (and never to > 10 g/dl). Exchange transfusions should only be for those who are severely unwell. HbSC is a milder variant with near normal haemoglobin. Prenatal diagnosis is possible after parental testing, using either CVS or amniocentesis.

Sickle cell trait

Heterozygotes who carry the HbS mutation on one chromosome 16 have this trait. There are no clinical problems in this condition, and indeed there is some protection against the effects of falciparum malarial infection. Forty percent of haemoglobin on electrophoresis is HbS, with HbA2 comprising 3% and the remainder being HbA1. The MCV and Hb are normal.

Disorders of globin synthesis

Thalassaemia results from a genetically determined imbalanced production of one of the globin chains. α-Thalassaemia affects α-globin chains whilst β-thalassaemia affects β-globin chains. α-Globin is coded for by two genes on chromosome 16, while β-globin is coded for by one gene on chromosome 11. Those with an MCV < 76 fl or MCH < 27 pg should be considered for further investigation. If positive, screen the other parent. There are many different genetic defects with differing prognoses and DNA analysis is important.

Never give parenteral iron.

β-Thalassaemia

β-Thalassaemia minor This is loss of function of one β-globin gene, with the tendency to anaemia corrected with oral $FeSO_4$ and folate. The HbA2 is 4–6%, with a slightly elevated HbF.

β-Thalassaemia major (Cooley's anaemia) Loss of function of two β-globin genes gives rise to this condition. There is increased iron uptake (despite excess iron stores), anaemia and progression to death without transfusions. There are also later problems with endocrine failure (including secondary sexual development), osteoporosis, haemosiderosis and cardiac failure. Transfusions suppress endogenous haemopoiesis, preventing skeletal deformity from marrow overgrowth (Hep C infection is now common). Consistent chelation therapy reduces problems of iron toxicity, and hydroxyurea is also used. Pregnancy may be possible following ovulation induction in those with good cardiac function. Marrow transplant is possible. The HbF is 50–100% on electrophoresis.

β-Thalassaemia

HbH disease This is loss of function of three α-globin genes. There is mild anaemia, the life expectancy is normal and treatment is with oral folate. β4 Tetramers form 5–30% of the haemoglobin on electrophoresis.

Bart's hydrops This is loss of all four α-globin genes. The hydropic fetus is non-viable, and the pregnancy is associated with an increased incidence of eclampsia and obstructed labour. Treatment is by termination of pregnancy.

LUNG DISORDERS

Pulmonary hypoplasia

This occurs most commonly as a consequence of oligohydramnios secondary to very preterm prelabour membrane rupture, Potter's syndrome (see p. 22), or diaphragmatic hernia (see below). Attempts to predict lung function based on linear measurements, chest circumference, lung volume or the presence of breathing movements have been disappointing.

Diaphragmatic hernia

Incidence 1:5000 LBs. Stomach, colon and even spleen enter the chest through a defect in the diaphragm, usually on the left. The heart is pushed to the right and the lungs become hypoplastic. The incidence of aneuploidy is 15–30% and there is an association with NTDs, CHD and renal and skeletal abnormalities. The overall survival of those diagnosed antenatally is ≈20%, with a better prognosis for isolated left-sided herniae (US Obstet Gynecol 1998:107). Polyhydramnios, mediastinal shift and left ventricular compression are poor antenatal prognostic factors. Increased nuchal translucency is also an adverse prognostic feature. For those who reach the stage of theatre, the survival rate is >80%. Neither the use of ECMO or nitric oxide has improved the prognosis. The chance of recurrence is approximately 2%, although there are occasional X-linked forms. New experimental therapeutic strategies include the use of a guided indwelling balloon to obstruct the fetal trachea in utero, allowing lung inflation and hernia reduction.

CCAM

This is a rare form of cystic lung disease. In types I and II there are multiple discernible thin-walled cysts; consideration may be given to antenatal aspiration if the cysts are large. In type III the cysts are very small and the lung appears large and hyperechoic (differentiate from bronchial obstruction and sequestration). The prognosis of this form is good in the absence of hydrops.

Bronchial cysts

These are rare.

SKELETAL DEFORMITIES

> There are over a hundred different syndromes, and it is often not possible to identify an individual one with certainty antenatally, or even occasionally postnatally. Often there is no family history of skeletal problems.

Nomenclature

Bone shortening may be distal (acromelia), proximal (rhizomelia) or overall shortened (micromelia). There may be complete absence of an extremity (amelia), or there may be an absent long bone with normal hand or foot (phocomelia). Clinodactyly describes overlapping digits, polydactyly extra digits, syndactyly fused digits and arthrogryphosis contractures of the extremities.

Ultrasound approach

Measure all long bones, assessing the degree and distribution of shortening. Also look at posture (abnormal posture suggests contractures) and for evidence of subtle hand and foot anomalies (which suggest abnormalities in other systems). Are there fractures or evidence of hypomineralization (usually indicating osteogenesis imperfecta)? Is the chest circumference small (suggestive, but not *indicative*, of lethal abnormality)? It is also important to look for extraskeletal abnormalities. The commonest dysplasias are listed in Table 1.4, but it is essential to consider a wider diagnostic list.

TABLE 1.4   Selected skeletal dysplasias

Syndrome	Epidemiology	Features
Thanatophoric dysplasia	1:10 000, sporadic, lethal	Severe micromelia, clover-leaf skull (14%), small chest, polyhydramnios (60%), flattened vertebral bodies, absent corpus callosum (20%)
Osteogenesis imperfecta, type I and IV	1:30 000, AD, usually non-lethal	Limb length normal, extremity bowing and reduced echogenicity may occur in late gestation. Different subtypes
Heterozygous achondroplasia	1:30 000, spontaneous mutation or AD, usually non-lethal	Progressive rhizomelic shortening beyond 24 weeks, large skull. (If homozygous, usually at least one parent affected, lethal. Features similar to thanatophoric dysplasia)
Achondrogenesis	1:40 000, AR, lethal	Severe micromelia, absent vertebral body ossification, poor skull ossification, occasional rib fractures, polyhydramnios
Osteogenesis imperfecta, type II	1:60 000, usually sporadic, lethal	Severe micromelia with deformity, apparent thickening of limb bones, diffuse hypomineralization allowing clear visualization of the sulci. The skull may be easily compressed. Multiple rib fractures with collapse of the rib cage. Different subtypes. Differentiate from congenital hypophosphataemia (also lethal)

Clinical management

As a precise antenatal diagnosis is often difficult, it is important to involve the parents and paediatricians in decision-making about method of delivery, intrapartum monitoring, appropriateness of intrapartum caesarean section and extent of postnatal resuscitation.

NON-IMMUNE HYDROPS   + PACE

There is skin oedema >5 mm and two or more of pericardial effusion, pleural effusion, ascites (Fig. 1.15) and a large placenta in the absence of antibody to red cell antigens (compare HDN, p. 43). The incidence is ≈1:2500 to 1:4000 LBs, and the mortality is 50–80%. There may be maternal problems in 80% due to polyhydramnios, pre-eclampsia or preterm labour. (POG 1993:33).

Causes

There are more than 100 recognized causes, most commonly those listed below.

Causes of non-immune hydrops

- Cardiovascular (structural anomalies including tachyarrhythmias and CHB (30%)
- Chromosomes (especially trisomies, Turner and triploidy) (15%)
- Infection (10%)
- Pulmonary abnormality (5%)
- Renal abnormality (3%)
- Structural abnormalities (diaphragmatic hernia, bladder neck obstruction), blood disorders (thalassaemias, G6PD deficiency) and placental or cord lesions are rare
- The remainder are rare

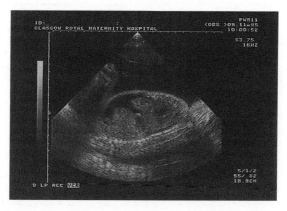

Fig. 1.15 Ascites at 20 weeks' gestation in non-immune hydrops fetalis.

Investigation is probably best carried out in a specialist fetal medicine unit:

- Is there a history of recent infections, or a family history of congenital disorders?
- Group, antibodies and Kleihauer–Betke stain.
- FBC ± electrophoresis for haemoglobinopathies.
- Viral titres for toxoplasmosis, CMV, rubella and human parvovirus B19.
- TPHA for syphilis.
- Autoantibody screen for anti-Ro, ANF and anti-DNA
- USS: detailed FA scan, including skeletal survey, echocardiography and Doppler.
- Amniocentesis for karyotype and culture; or FBS (only if >22 weeks) for FBC, blood group and direct Coombs test, karyotype, viral serology and haemoglobin electrophoresis.

Management

- If there is a dysrhythmia, see page 13.
- Intrauterine transfusions of RCC may be of value in some cases, especially in parvovirus B19.
- Draining serous cavities (particularly the pleural cavity) under ultrasound guidance may be helpful, but fluid accumulates within 48 hours.
- Avoid delivery before term if possible.
- Delivery by caesarean section does not affect outcome, but allows planned paediatric care.
- Consider termination of pregnancy (and postmortem) if very preterm.

Mun do not recur .

OTHER INHERITED CONDITIONS

α_1-antitrypsin deficiency (AR)
There are more than 75 genetic variants, most of which are benign. One case in 3000 is homozygous for the PiZ gene, and about 30% will present with infantile hepatitis, which can progress to cirrhosis. A further 30% will develop early or midlife emphysema. The antenatal diagnosis of PiZ is possible using DNA from amniocentesis or CVS.

Albinism (AR but some AD or X-linked)
Incidence 1:20 000 LBs. There are at least 10 types.

Congenital adrenal hyperplasia (AR)
Incidence 1:10 000 LBs. There is usually a 21-hydroxylase deficiency, which presents with ambiguous genitalia in a female fetus or with macrogenitosomia in the male. Antenatal diagnosis is possible with CVS (see also Ambiguous Genitalia, p. 173).

Beckwith–Weidmann syndrome

This is characterized by a large tongue and kidneys with exomphalos (often small) and microcephaly. There are early feeding difficulties.

Cystic fibrosis (AR)

The UK gene frequency is 1:25 (i.e. heterozygote frequency), giving an estimated overall couple risk for a live birth of around 1:2500. Clinically, there is respiratory, gastrointestinal, liver and pancreatic dysfunction, and azoospermia is the rule. The prognosis is very variable and although death in the age group 20–30 years still occurs, the prognosis is improving and many now live considerably longer. The health of an affected sibling is not a prognostic guide to the health of other siblings. Four mutant alleles account for 85% of the gene defects in the UK (the commonest being ΔF508), and antenatal screening for these is possible using saliva specimens, with CVS being performed if both parents are gene carriers (see also p. 144).

Cystic hygroma (MF)

Cystic hygromas probably develop from a defect in the formation of lymphatic vessels – it is likely that the lymphatic system and venous system fail to connect and lymph fluid accumulates in the jugular lymph sacs. Larger hygromas are frequently divided by septae. Check also for skin oedema, ascites, pleural and pericardial effusions, and cardiac and renal abnormalities. There is an association with aneuploidy (particularly Turner's, Down's and Edward's syndromes) and it is appropriate to offer karyotyping. If generalized hydrops is present the prognosis is bleak. Isolated hygromas may be surgically corrected postnatally and have a good prognosis. Only rarely are they so large as to result in dystocia.

Facial clefts (MF)

Incidence 1:1000 LBs. These are mostly idiopathic, but are occasionally associated with rare single gene defects or chromosomal abnormalities (e.g. T13 or T18). There is also an association with benzodiazepine use, folate acid antagonists and rubella. There are other structural malformations in 15–50% of cases. Repair of unilateral or incomplete lesions gives good cosmetic results, but there is often some residual deformity with bilateral lesions. Avoid taking the baby to the SCBU if possible (to aid bonding). The risk of recurrence of isolated lesions (with normal parents) is 1:50 for unilateral defects and 1:20 for bilateral defects. Isolated cleft palate occurs in 1:2500 births and carries a recurrence risk of 1:50 for both siblings and offspring. Midline clefts are rare, and holoprosencephaly should be excluded.

Fragile X syndrome (XL)

Incidence 0.7:1000 male LBs, 0.4:1000 female LBs. This is the commonest cause of moderate mental retardation after Down's syndrome and the commonest form of inherited mental handicap. Males are usually more severely affected than females. Speech delay is common and there is an associated behavioural phenotype, with gaze aversion. The condition is caused by the expansion of a CGG triplet repeat on the X chromosome. Normal individuals have an average of 29 repeats, but for an unexplained reason this may increase to a premutation of 50–200 repeats. Those with a premutation are phenotypically normal, but the premutation is unstable during female meiosis and can expand to a full mutation of more than 200 repeats. There is an approximately 10% chance of this occurring (in the absence of a full mutation in that generation already). This causes the fragile X phenotype in 99% of males and in around 30–50% of females. Parental screening is possible and CVS may be used to identify the degree of amplification of the CGG repeats in potential offspring. (For other repeat disorders see Myotonic Dystrophy and Huntington's Chorea, below.)

Galactosaemia (AR)
Incidence 1:200 000 LBs. This transferase deficiency is usually fatal before 4 weeks of life due to cachexia and septicaemia. A lactose-free diet is essential, and recent reports have suggested that mild learning difficulties and infertility can be associated with the condition even if a strict diet is followed. Antenatal diagnosis is possible.

Haemophilia

Haemophilia A (XL) Incidence 0.2:1000 male LBs. There is deficiency of factor VIII. Antenatal diagnosis may be possible with specific markers or known factor VIII mutations.

Haemophilia B (XL) Incidence 0.03:1000 male LBs. There is deficiency of factor IX. Antenatal diagnosis may be possible.

Haemorrhagic disease of the newborn
HDN results from a lack of vitamin K (there are no enteric bacteria) and presents with systemic bleeding. The classical form occurs between days 1 and 7, although an early form occurs in infants born to mothers taking anticonvulsants, and a late (and sometimes more serious) form may also occur. Almost complete protection is given by the administration of vitamin K (1 mg IM) at the time of birth, and possibly less complete protection is provided by giving vitamin K (2 mg PO) twice in the first week (with a further oral dose at 1 month). Some epidemiological studies have found an association between IM vitamin K (as opposed to oral) and childhood leukaemias, resulting in a swing away from treatment. Two subsequent studies (N Engl J Med 1993;329:905 and Br Med J 1993;307:89) involving 1.25 million children and 48 cases of malignancy have failed to prove the connection.

Hirschsprung's disease (MF)

Incidence 1:8000 LBs with a 3:1 male excess. If the child is male, the chance of sibling recurrence is 1:25. If female, this chance is 1:8. The risk of recurrence if one or other parent has been affected is <1:100.

Huntington's chorea (AD)

Incidence 4–560:100 000 LBs. The onset usually occurs after the age of 30, although it may present as early as 10–15 years of age. There is dementia, mood change (usually depression) and choreoathetosis progressing to death in approximately 15 years. There is a CAG trinucleotide expansion on chromosome 4p, allowing accurate carrier and prenatal testing. (For other repeat disorders see Fragile X Syndrome, above, and Myotonic Dystrophy, below.)

Hurler's mucopolysaccharidosis (AR)

Incidence 1:40 000 LBs. This disease is fatal between 5 and 10 years of age. Antenatal diagnosis is possible.

Marfan's syndrome (AD)

Incidence 1:20 000 LBs. The individual is tall, doliocephalic and carries the risk of kyphoscoliosis, ectopia lentis, aortic regurgitation and dissecting aortic aneurysm. One in 10 individuals with Marfan's syndrome has a dilated aortic root and prophylactic β blockade is recommended. Aortic-root diameter should be monitored during the pregnancy of a woman with Marfan's syndrome.

Muscular dystrophy

This refers to a group of primary muscle-wasting diseases which are genetically determined and usually progressive.

Becker muscular dystrophy (XL recessive) This is also caused by mutations (usually in-frame deletions) in the dystrophin gene. Intellectual impairment is less common and the progression is slower than with Duchenne muscular dystrophy. The two disorders can be differentiated by dystrophin analysis on muscle biopsy.

Congenital muscular dystrophy This refers to several distinct diseases, usually with AR inheritance, presenting with a floppy infant ± arthrogryphosis and contractures. The prognosis is very variable, but often good.

Duchenne muscular dystrophy (XL recessive) Incidence 0.3:1000 males. It is caused by mutations in the dystrophin gene. There is occasional mild intellectual impairment in 30%, and progressive muscle weakness such that the patient is usually wheelchair dependent by 10–12 years of age; 75% die before 20 years; 95% by 50 years. There may also be an associated cardiomyopathy. Two-thirds of affected boys are carriers, one-third representing new mutations. Antenatal diagnosis with CVS is possible in the 70% of families, where the dystrophin gene mutation is readily detected if the family structure is suitable for linkage analysis.

Facioscapulohumeral muscular dystrophy (often AD) There is shoulder weakness, usually coming on around 12–14 years, associated with difficulty sucking and whistling. It is usually relatively benign, but there is marked familial variation.

Limb girdle muscular dystrophy (AR) There is progressive weakness usually beginning in early adult life and often requiring a wheelchair by the age of 30.

Myotonia congenita (Thomsen's disease) (AD)
There is a non-progressive myotonia and failure to relax the grasp. Intelligence is normal.

Myotonic dystrophy (AD)
This condition characteristically presents in early or mid-adult life and is caused by the expansion of a CTG triplet repeat on chromosome 19. The degree of expansion correlates with severity of presentation, being largest in babies with congenital onset. There is grip and percussion myotonia with muscle weakness, particularly of proximal muscles. Other features include early cataracts and premature frontal balding. Women who have symptomatic disease are at particular risk of conceiving infants with congenital myotonic dystrophy. In this condition there is a high pregnancy loss rate, and both polyhydramnios and premature labour are common. Infants are born floppy and make little or no respiratory effort. Talipes and feeding difficulties are frequently encountered and, if the infant survives, learning difficulties and severe constipation are regular findings. A significant proportion die before 3 months of age. Antenatal diagnosis is possible using DNA from CVS or amniocentesis. (For other repeat disorders see Fragile X Syndrome, p. 28, and Huntington's Chorea, p. 30).

Neurofibromatosis type 1 (AD)
Incidence 1:2500 LBs. Café au lait patches are found on the skin and neurofibromas develop on peripheral nerve sheaths (the risk of malignancy is about 6%). The neurofibromas may be removed surgically. The condition can also be associated with phaeochromocytomas and renal artery stenosis. One in 10 gene carriers has learning difficulties.

Phenylketonuria (AR)
Incidence 1:15000 LBs. There is a deficiency of the enzyme phenylalanine hydroxylase leading to a low level of tyrosine and a high, toxic level of phenylalanine. This leads to convulsions and mental retardation if untreated. Management is by giving a phenylalanine free diet. In pregnancy, the

phenylalanine level should remain less than at least 500 μmol/l (but ideally 50–150 μmol/l) to minimize risks of IUGR, mental retardation and CHD (especially Fallot's tetralogy). There should also be tyrosine supplementation (aiming to maintain the tyrosine level at 60–90 μmol/l).

Radiation

Fetal doses resulting from most conventional diagnostic procedures have no increased association with fetal death, malformation or the impairment of fetal development. The threshold dose above which there are risks of gross malformation or fetal demise is 250–500 mGy at <8 weeks' gestation. After 8 weeks, gross malformations are only rarely seen, but the threshold for demise up to 20 weeks is >500 mGy, and from then until term it is >1000 mGy. The risk of mental retardation is probably negligible both before 8 weeks and beyond 25 weeks, and there is probably no effect between 15 and 25 weeks with doses of <500 mGy. There may be a very small dose-related association with mental retardation at 8–15 weeks. The risk of radiation-induced genetic disease in descendants of the unborn child is unknown, but there are no human data to suggest a risk, and there is no indication for TOP or the use of invasive investigations (e.g. amniocentesis). The risk of inducing childhood cancer is small at around 1:17 000 per mGy (baseline risk 1:650 per mGy). A CXR exposes the fetus to <0.01 mGy, a pelvis view to 1.1 mGy, an IVU to 1.7 mGy, a ^{99m}Tc lung scan to 0.2 mGy, a CT of the head to <0.005 mGy, and a pelvic CT to 25 mGy (although the exposure from CT pelvimetry is only 0.2 mGy) (National Radiological Protection Board 1998).

Spherocytosis (AD)

There is variable expression, which may include jaundice, anaemia and splenomegaly. Treatment is with splenectomy at between 5 and 10 years of age. Antenatal diagnosis is possible.

Tay–Sachs disease (AR)

The gene frequency is 1:30 in Ashkenazi Jews, but is rare in other groups. There is a build up of gangliosides within the CNS leading to retardation, paralysis and blindness. By the age of 4 years, the child is usually dead or in a vegetative state. Carriers may be screened by measuring the level of hexosaminidase A in leukocytes.

Teratomas (MF)

These are usually sacrococcygeal and are treatable in early neonatal life with surgery. Hydrops may develop in the second trimester secondary to arteriovenous shunting. However, 10–30% are malignant and, although these are indistinguishable from the benign form on USS, the prognosis following chemotherapy is good. Delivery is usually by caesarean section on account of the size of the tumour. There are numerous other rare soft-tissue cysts or tumours which may occur at different sites.

Tuberous sclerosis (AD)

Incidence 1:50 000 LBs. There are gliomas, which only very rarely become malignant. The clinical presentation is with infantile spasms and mental retardation from birth. In 30% of cases there are also rhabdomyomas. Antenatal diagnosis with CVS or amniocentesis is possible.

Umbilical artery (MF)

A single umbilical artery in the third trimester is associated with abnormality in 50% of fetuses, particularly of the urinary tract, heart, gastrointestinal system and ear. There is an 8–60% association with aneuploidy and a 10–20% association with IUGR.

Von Willebrand disease (AD)

This is due to a deficiency of factor VIII carrier protein and manifests as platelet disorder (e.g. bleeding after surgery). Diagnosis is made by demonstrating reduced platelet aggregation with ristocetin. Antenatal diagnosis is possible.

VATER association

This refers to a condition in which there are vertebral, anal, tracheal or esophageal and renal lesions. (Also, extended to VACTERL by adding cardiac and limb abnormalities.)

DRUGS IN PREGNANCY (Table 1.5)

> See The British National Formulary, Appendices 4 and 5 (new editions 6 monthly) and Br Med J 1998;317:1503.

The statement that all drugs are potential teratogens may seem harsh, but it emphasizes that one can never confirm the safety of any drug in pregnancy. One can only report on problems that seem to have arisen. As a general principle, all drugs should be avoided in pregnancy unless clinical benefits are likely to outweigh the risks to the fetus. A useful treatment, however, should not be stopped without good reason.

The major body structures are formed in about the first 12 weeks or so and drug treatment before this time may cause a teratogenic effect. If a drug is given after this time it will not produce a major anatomical defect, but may affect the growth and development of the baby.

TABLE 1.5   Drugs in pregnancy

Class of drug	Drug	Risk to fetus
Local anaesthetics	Prilocaine	Methaemoglobinaemia may occur if used in epidural infusions. Use lignocaine or bupivacaine instead
General anaesthetics	All agents	Any risks are probably related to large doses of barbiturates for induction and to the possible teratogenic risks of hypoxia itself. There is some animal evidence to suggest an increased risk of abortion after exposure to anaesthetic gases, although there is no evidence that the abortion rate is greater in exposed theatre personnel
Analgesics	Aspirin	There were no significant problems associated with low-dose aspirin use in the Collaborative Low Dose Aspirin Study in Pregnancy (CLASP) report (Lancet 1994;343:619). Analgesic doses may lead to impaired platelet function and an increased risk of haemorrhage
	Indomethacin and other PG inhibitors	Cause impairment of renal function and may lead to premature closure of the ductus arteriosis. There may also be an association with persistent pulmonary hypertension in the newborn
	Opiates/opioids	See page 119
	Paracetamol	Thought to be safe for use in pregnancy
Antacids and ulcer-healing drugs	Alkalis	Retrospective studies have suggested a slightly increased incidence of congenital abnormalities in children born to mothers receiving antacids during the first 56 days of pregnancy. This is not confirmed in available prospective studies
	Cimetidine	Avoid, as may have antiandrogenic effects
	Omeprazole	Toxicity in animal studies. Avoid
	Ranitidine	No known problems
Antiarrhythmics	Amiodarone	Theoretical risk of depressing fetal thyroid. Avoid
Antibiotics	Aminoglycosides	There is a risk of fetal ototoxicity. Monitor levels.
	Chloramphenicol	The risk of 'grey-baby syndrome' from use around term is small
	Co-trimoxazole	The sulpha component may displace bilirubin and cause kernicterus. There is also some evidence of teratogenesis (trimethoprim is a folate antagonist). Both components should be avoided in pregnancy
	Erythromycin base	Thought to be safe for use in pregnancy
	Fluconazole	Toxicity at high doses in animal studies. Avoid use in pregnancy
	Fluoroquinolones (e.g. ciprofloxacin)	These cause arthropathy in animal studies. Norfloxacin has also been shown to be embryocidal in animal studies. Avoid.

	Metronidazole	There is growing evidence to support its safety in pregnancy
	Penicillins	Thought to be safe for use in pregnancy
	Tetracyclines	Contraindicated in pregnancy, as they become permanently incorporated into growing bones and deciduous teeth, leading to discolouration. Affect skeletal development in animal studies only. Avoid
Anticoagulants	Warfarin and heparin	See page 146
Anticonvulsants (see also p. 122)	Carbamazepine	There is a risk of craniofacial defects, neural tube defects and developmental delay. There is also a risk of neonatal haemorrhage – give maternal vitamin K in late pregnancy and neonatal vitamin K at birth (see p. 122)
	Gabapentin, lamotrigine and vigabatrin	Data remain limited. Animal studies suggest that gabapentin and lamotrigine are relatively safe, but vigabatrin has teratogenic properties
	Phenobarbitone	There may be teratogenic problems. There is a risk of neonatal haemorrhage – give maternal vitamin K in late pregnancy and neonatal vitamin K at birth (see p. 122)
	Phenytoin	There may be teratogenic problems, particularly cardiac abnormalities, mental retardation, craniofacial defects and diaphragmatic herniae. Serum folate levels may be lowered, so maternal folate supplements are warranted. There is also a risk of neonatal haemorrhage – give maternal vitamin K in late pregnancy and neonatal vitamin K at birth (see p. 122)
	Primadone	As for phenytoin
	Sodium valproate	There is an increase in the incidence of neural tube defects, microcephaly and cardiac abnormalities. Give folic acid preconception or as soon as possible in the first trimester (see p. 122)
Antidepressants	MAOIs	Very limited data suggest risk of malformations. Avoid in all stages of pregnancy
	Lithium	Exposure in the first trimester has been linked with congenital heart disease. Neonatal goitre, hypotonia, cyanosis, lethargy and cardiac arrhythmias have resulted from later transplacental exposure. Avoid if possible but, if used, monitor serum levels closely
	SSRIs	No evidence of teratogenicity in humans, but data are limited. There is evidence of animal teratogenicity. Only use if benefits outweigh risks
	Tricyclic antidepressants	The risks are low and there has been more experience with tricyclics in pregnancy than with other antidepressants. May lead to neonatal tachycardia, irritability and muscle spasms

Anti-hypertensives	ACE inhibitors	May adversely affect fetal BP, and renal function in fetus and newborn. Also, possible skull defects. Avoid
	Methyl-dopa	This is widely used and is thought to be safe, although there are reports of ileus with very high doses. There may be a false-positive Coombs test in the fetus
	β Blockers	Possible association with IUGR, and more definite associations with neonatal bradycardia and neonatal hypoglycaemia
	Prochlorperazine	Uncertain teratogenesis
Antihistamines	Chlorpheniramine, terfenadine	Chlorpheniramine is thought to be safe in pregnancy. There is little experience with the newer preparations
Antimalarials	All preparations	For prophylaxis, chloroquine is preferred. In treatment of malarial infection, benefits far outweigh the risks
Antimitotics	Idoxuridine	There is evidence of animal teratogenesis. Avoid
	Podophyllin	There are reports of teratogenesis and fetal death after topical wart treatment. Avoid
Antipsychotics	Chlorpromazine and related phenothiazines	No consistent teratogenic effect has been demonstrated. If antipsychotic drugs are required, chlorpromazine and trifluoperazine are probably the ones of choice. Extrapyramidal effects are occasionally seen in the neonate. There is a relatively higher incidence of problems with depot preparations
	Haloperidol	There are several poorly documented reports of limb-reduction deformities. Extrapyramidal reactions in the newborn have been described
Antithyroid drugs (see also p. 150)	Carbimazole, propylthiouracil	May cause neonatal hypothyroidism
Antivirals	Aciclovir	Experience small; use only when benefits outweigh risks. There is only limited absorption from topical preparations
Bronchodilators	Aminophylline	Causes neonatal apnoea and irritability
	Inhaled preparations	All inhaled preparations, including inhaled steroids, are considered safe in pregnancy
Diuretics	Thiazides	First-trimester exposure may cause an increased risk of congenital defects. Neonatal thrombocytopenia and hypoglycaemia may occur if used near term. Avoid
	Frusemide	May lead to reduced placental perfusion. Avoid
Hypoglycaemics	Chlorpropamide, tolbutamide	May cause neonatal hypoglycaemia
Iron supplements	Many preparations	Thought to be safe

Retinoids	Etretinate, isotretinoin	High risk of fetal malformation sufficient to consider TOP. Contraception should be used from 1 month before to at least 2 years after stopping treatment. Also avoid topical treatment
Sedatives/ tranquillizers	Benzodiazepines	See page 119
Sex hormones	Androgens (including danazol)	Small risk of causing masculinization of a female fetus. Avoid
	Oestrogens	May cause urogenital defects in a male fetus. Stilboestrol is associated with later vaginal adenocarcinoma. Avoid
	Progestogens	May cause masculinisation of a female fetus. Avoid
	Combined oral contraceptive	Meta-analysis does not support any evidence of teratogenesis (Obstet Gynecol 1995;85:141)
Steroids		Although there are associations with fetal abnormality in animal studies, particularly cleft palate, there have been no teratogenic effects demonstrated in humans, despite extensive usage. Fetal adrenal suppression possible with >10 mg/day prednisolone
Vaccines		There is a theoretical risk of teratogenic problems from vaccines. In principle only, live vaccines (BCG, MMR, oral polio, oral typhoid, yellow fever) should be avoided if possible. Nonetheless, for any vaccine, the protective benefits probably outweigh any potential risks
Vitamins	A	Excessive doses in the first trimester may be teratogenic
	D	There may be a risk of skeletal abnormalities in high-dose regimens

ANTENATAL PROBLEMS

BREECH PRESENTATION

> The incidence of breech presentation is 40% at 20 weeks, 25% at 32 weeks and 3% at term. The chance of spontaneous version after 38 weeks is less than 4%. It is associated with multiple pregnancy, bicornuate uterus, fibroids, placenta praevia, polyhydramnios and oligohydramnios. It is also associated with fetal anomaly (approximately three times more commonly than in the cephalic population) particularly NTDs, neuromuscular disorders and autosomal trisomies. The incidence of lethal malformations in an *unscreened* population is ≈8:1000 (compared with ≈1.5:1000 in those with cephalic presentation). At term, 65% of breech presentations are frank (extended). The remainder are flexed or footling (the latter carries a 5–20% risk of cord prolapse).

There is no firm evidence to recommend elective caesarean section over planned selected vaginal delivery for breech presentation at term (Br J Obstet Gynaecol 1998:710). The risk of intrapartum caesarean section during a planned vaginal delivery is about 30%.

OPTIONS

External cephalic version

This should be carried out at ≈38 week. It is contraindicated with placenta praevia, multiple pregnancy, and APH, and relatively contraindicated in those with pre-eclampsia, IUGR and a previous caesarean section. Check a CTG and ultrasound. Some obstetricians like the patient to be fasted and prepared for theatre. Although this is usually not necessary, it is reasonable to have access to theatre close at hand. It is most likely to be successful when the presenting part is free, the head is easy to palpate and the uterus feels soft (Br J Obstet Gynaecol 1997:798).

Ask the mother to lie flat with a 30° lateral tilt. If the uterus is not soft, establish a ritodrine IV infusion at 200 µg/min for 15 minutes (see p. 71). Scanning gel allows easier manipulation and permits scanning during the procedure, if required. Disengage the breech with the scan probe or hands, and then attempt to rotate in the direction in which the baby is facing (i.e. forward roll/somersault). Check the FH every 2 minutes. If unsuccessful, return to breech rather than leave transverse. Give anti-D (500 IU IM) if rhesus negative. The success rate of version is ≈30% for primigravidae and ≈50% for parous women.

Vaginal delivery (for delivery technique, see p. 84)

This may be appropriate if the estimated fetal weight is <3.8 kg with no fetal compromise, pre-eclampsia or placenta praevia. Ideally the onset of labour should be spontaneous, the breech frank or flexed (but not footling) and the liquor volume normal. Radiographic pelvimetry is recommended. The incidence of caesarean section in those planning a vaginal breech delivery in the UK is approximately 50%. The risk of serious intrapartum fetal problems is low, probably less than 1% (Am J Obstet Gynecol 1980;137(2):235, Am J Obstet Gynecol 1983;146(1):34). Potential problems include intracranial injury, widespread bruising, damage to internal organs, spinal cord transection, umbilical cord prolapse and hypoxia following obstruction of the after-coming head. Those not assessed antenatally and presenting in advanced labour with an engaged breech usually deliver without adverse consequences (Br J Obstet Gynaecol 1993:531).

Caesarean section

There is increased maternal morbidity and mortality over vaginal delivery from pulmonary embolism, infection, anaesthetic problems, psychological problems and bladder or bowel injury. The operation is usually safe for the baby, but can be very traumatic in extreme prematurity (a De Lees or classical incision may help) and should be performed by an experienced obstetrician. Also bear in mind that the risk of uterine dehiscence in subsequent labours is ≈1%. It is probably advisable to carry out a caesarean section if the estimated fetal weight is <1500 g or the gestation is <32 weeks, as there is a risk of the cervix closing around the neck after delivery of the breech (Br J Obstet Gynaecol 1993:411).

Remember

Check all babies presenting by the breech for CDH and Klumpke's paralysis.

FETAL MONITORING (ANTENATAL)

Antenatal monitoring is used in the hope of identifying fetal compromise in utero. Resist the temptation to act on one abnormality when all else seems normal if the risks to the fetus of an early delivery are high. It is always essential to assess the complete clinical picture when considering the results of investigations, particularly the previous obstetric history, medical history, fetal growth, movements and other investigations.

Fetal movement

These are used as a screening test for further investigations. The patient is often asked to choose a starting time (usually 9 a.m.) and record how long it takes to feel 10 separate movements. If there have been <10 movements by, say, 5 p.m. she is asked to contact for further tests (e.g. CTG). There is great variation in what may be considered as normal, and 'a change in the usual movements' may be more important than absolute numbers.

Cardiotocograph

The interpretation of CTGs is discussed on page 74. Unprovoked decelerations (i.e. in the absence of contractions) occur in ≈8% of normal pre-term traces, and interpretation of these depends on the character of the remainder of the CTG (particularly variability and accelerations). Decelerations *may* be physiological at earlier gestations. The CTG gives an indication of fetal well-being at that given moment but has little longer term value.

Doppler

Doppler ultrasound of the umbilical arteries is used as an assessment of downstream vascular (placental) resistance (US Obstet Gynecol 1997:271). Reduction or loss of end-diastolic flow identifies the fetus at high risk of hypoxia, and indeed this hypoxia probably precedes Doppler abnormalities. A normal Doppler study, therefore, does not exclude hypoxia and tests of fetal well-being (e.g. CTG and amniotic fluid volume) must also be employed for complete assessment. There is probably no useful screening role for routine Doppler studies in low-risk pregnancies.

Umbilical artery Doppler is useful in pregnancies considered at risk of hypoxia due to impaired placental function. In particular, a normal waveform would indicate that a SGA fetus was constitutionally small rather than growth restricted due to impaired placental function (Br Med J 1990;300:1044). Abnormal waveforms are associated with an increased risk of structural and chromosomal abnormalities, and detailed sonography is indicated to avoid inappropriate iatrogenic morbidity (Obstet Gynecol 1991;77:374).

Doppler studies of the maternal uterine arteries at 20–24 weeks may be useful in high-risk pregnancies (essential hypertension, a history of pre-eclampsia, 'unexplained' raised αFP) to identify the presence of bilateral notching or high-resistance flow (about 5% of pregnancies). Patients with persistent bilateral notching (i.e. >24 weeks) are particularly at risk of developing pre-eclampsia (sensitivity >70%, PPV 27% in an unselected population) and delivering a SGA fetus (sensitivity 57%, PPV 31%). Only 1% of women will develop pre-eclampsia with a normal uterine artery Doppler study (US Obstet Gynecol 1996:182).

Biophysical profile

Five parameters are assessed, scored as 2 each, and the total out of 10 used to give an indication of fetal well-being (Table 2.1) (Obstet Gynecol 1984;64:326). Of all the parameters, liquor volume is probably the most predictive of fetal well-being. The CTG may be considered separately (and the score therefore given out of 8). Although available for many years the score is time consuming and there is little evidence of benefit over the non-stress CTG or Doppler (Br J Obstet Gynaecol 1990;97:909).

TABLE 2.1   Parameters of the biophysical profile

CTG	More than 2 accelerations of 15 bpm lasting longer than 15 s in 20 min
Fetal breathing	Lasting more than 30 s in 30 min
Fetal movements	More than 3 limb or trunk movements in 30 min
Fetal tone	One return to flexion (of neck) after extension, or one hand opening and closing
Liquor volume	More than 3 cm depth in 2 planes

HAEMOLYTIC DISEASE OF THE NEWBORN

Maternal IgG antibodies to fetal red cell antigens cross the placenta and cause fetal haemolysis, anaemia and hydrops fetalis. Initial sensitization usually occurs at delivery, but may also occur with PV bleeding at any stage, amniocentesis, ECV or at some unrecognized event (10% of affected pregnancies). It tends to become more severe with subsequent pregnancies: if the last baby died from rhesus haemolytic disease the chance of successful outcome in the next pregnancy is <50%. There are >700 known antigens, but rhesus accounts for more than 95% of haemolytic disease.

PROPHYLAXIS

Prophylaxis is only available for the 'D' antigen. It is available in 250, 500, 2500 and 5000 IU/vial. A dose of 125 IU is sufficient to react with 1–2 ml of fetal blood.

Antenatal
Anti-D should be given to Rhesus-negative mothers following any PV bleeding in pregnancy (including ectopic, abortion, CVS, amniocentesis, cordocentesis, ECV, external trauma and APH).

- If <20 weeks, give 250 IU IM stat.
- If >20 weeks, give an initial 500 IU IM stat. and carry out a Kleihauer test (estimates the volume of fetal blood transfused). Give more anti-D if indicated by the Kleihauer result.
- If there is ongoing intermittent bleeding, repeat the anti-D 6-weekly.

Prophylaxis is likely to be more effective if anti-D is given to all Rhesus-negative mothers routinely in the third trimester (either 500 IU at 28 and 34 weeks, or a single larger dose early in the third trimester). This is not currently standard practice in the UK, in part due to insufficient polyvalent anti-D supply (Br J Obstet Gynaecol 1998: 129) but this situation is changing at the time of going to press.

Postnatal

If mother is Rhesus negative and the baby Rhesus positive, check a Kleihauer test and give an initial 500 IU anti-D IM stat. More anti-D may be required following the Kleihauer result. The anti-D should be administered within 72 hours.

SCREENING

Approximately 15% of women in the UK are Rhesus negative. All women should be screened for all antibodies at booking. The maternal serum level of the antibody (usually anti-D) is used as an initial screening test for further action. There are regional variations, but an example of when to check levels is shown in Table 2.2 (Transfusion Med 1994;6:71).

TABLE 2.2 Potential screening programme for antibodies in haemolytic disease of the newborn

All pregnant women (including RhD +ve)	ABO + RhD group and antibody screen	At 10–16 weeks
	Rh D group and antibody screen	At 28–36 weeks
Patients with autoantibodies		
Anti-D, c or Kell related	Antibody screen/titre	At least monthly to 28 weeks, then 2 weekly to term
Other antibodies	Antibody screen/titre	At 28–36 weeks, thereafter on titre, etc.

RHESUS DISEASE

Without recourse to prophylaxis, 1% of Rhesus-negative mothers would develop anti-D in their first pregnancy and 3–5% in subsequent pregnancies. If antibody is detected, check the paternal genotype. If the father is homozygous for 'd', then both he and the fetus will be Rhesus negative, making significant Rhesus disease unlikely. If heterozygous for 'D', there is a 50% chance that the fetus will be Rhesus positive and if homozygous, the chance is 100%. Those mothers with rising antibody levels are sometimes assessed by amniocentesis as outlined below. It is probably more appropriate, however, to refer them to a specialist fetal medicine unit for fetal blood sampling. If the previous pregnancy has been complicated by Rhesus iso-immunization, perform the first invasive investigation 10 weeks before the previous intrauterine death, intrauterine transfusion or delivery. Also consider investigations with a rising level of maternal antibody level, or if there are reduced fetal movements, or if there is ultrasound evidence of fetal anaemia (e.g. ascites, cardiomegaly, pleural effusions or polyhydramnios). Severe disease is rare if the maternal antibody is <4 IU/ml. The risk of severe disease is moderate if maternal antibody is 4–15 IU/ml, and there is a risk of severe anaemia in 50% of fetuses when the level is >15 IU/ml.

Amniocentesis

This is carried out to measure amniotic fluid bilirubin levels with spectrophotometry at OD_{450} (note that artefactual levels occur following chronic maternal steroid administration). The result is plotted on a Liley chart to decide between conservative management, intrauterine transfusion or delivery. There is evidence, however, that serum levels of anti-D correlate so well with amniocentesis findings that amniocentesis is not necessary, fetal blood sampling being preferable (Br J Obstet Gynaecol 1993:923).

Fetal blood sampling

This is carried out under ultrasound guidance. The blood group can be checked and, if the haematocrit (or in some centres haemoglobin) is low, the fetus is transfused with a calculated volume of group O Rhesus-negative blood which has been cross-matched to the mother's own serum. The transfusion may be given intraperitoneally or by the intravascular route. Fetal blood sampling carries the risk of cord haematoma, bradycardia, intrauterine death and further sensitization of the mother to fetal red cell antigens. It is usually repeated again every 2 weeks and delivery performed around 36 weeks.

OTHER ANTIBODIES

Other antigens

Many of these (e.g. anti-c, Kell, e, Ce, Fy^a, Jk^a, C^w) are poorly developed on the red cell surface and usually stimulate only low levels of antibody production, often of the IgM category (which does not cross the placenta). Some will, however, cause significant HDN. Note particularly that anti-Kell causes marrow aplasia rather than HDN, and therefore serum antibody levels and the OD_{450} are poor predictors of disease severity. It is important to check the paternal genotype to assess the risk of anti-Kell disease and FBS must be used to assess disease severity. The inheritance is AD, the gene being called K (most people are 'k' positive, also termed 'cellano' positive). Anti-Le^a, Le^b, Lu^a, P, N, Xg^a and Kn^a have not been associated with HDN (Br J Obstet Gynaecol;1996:195).

Du antigen → does not form AntiD → ∴ does not require Anti D (RCOG guideline)

Treat as Rhesus negative for the purposes of haemolytic disease of the newborn.

ABO

In 15% of pregnancies the mother will be group O and the fetus A or B. This rarely causes significant HDN and the risk to the fetus is very low. The severity in subsequent pregnancies is unpredictable owing to the variability of red cell protein expression. ABO incompatibility in Rhesus-negative mothers very much reduces the likelihood of Rhesus iso-immunization to a Rhesus-positive fetus. No antenatal investigations are warranted.

HYPEREMESIS GRAVIDARUM

Nausea and vomiting occur in 50–80% of pregnancies in the first trimester. Inability to keep down fluids or solids leads to weight loss (2 to >5 kg), dehydration, electrolyte disturbances and vitamin B deficiency (polyneuropathy), and may very rarely lead to liver failure, renal failure and fetal or maternal death. (Br J Obstet Gynaecol 1993;8:708).

Check

- U&E, haematocrit, MSU, urine for ketones and TFTs (see Hyperthyroidism, p. 150).
- LFTs if severe or prolonged (↓albumin, ↑transaminases, PTR normal).
- USS: ? multiple pregnancy or hydatidiform mole.
- Social aspects of admission.

Treatment

Admission and IV fluids are usually sufficient by themselves to reduce nausea and should be the only initial management. The patient should eat a little often. Antiemetics may be used only if the vomiting is not settling. No antiemetics are licensed for use in pregnancy. There is an unquantified, but probably very low, risk of teratogenesis:

- metoclopramide 10 mg IM/IV TID;
- cyclizine 50 mg IM/IV TID;
- domperidone 30 mg suppository PR QID;
- prochlorperazine 12.5 mg IM TID;
- chlorpromazine 100 mg suppository QID (may lead to jaundice and extrapyramidal side-effects in the fetus).

If the vomiting is prolonged, severe and unresponsive to standard management, consider prednisolone 20 mg PO BD or TID or ondansetron 8 mg PO BD or 16 mg/day PR. Also consider enteral feeding (or TPN) and vitamin B supplementation. Abnormal LFTs respond rapidly to correction of dehydration and malnutrition.

EATING DISORDERS

The incidence of bulimia and anorexia nervosa in pregnancy is less than in the non-pregnant population.

Bulimia

Bulimics tend to improve in later pregnancy and often become worse again after delivery. There may be a slightly greater incidence of fetal anomaly.

Anorexia nervosa

Anorexics may become worse as pregnancy advances. The incidence of low-birth-weight infants is increased, particularly if ovulation induction has been used to assist conception. The perinatal mortality is also greater. Delay ovulation induction until the weight is >45 kg.

INTRAUTERINE DEATH

> This is defined as intrauterine death after 24 weeks' gestation. If left alone, 80% will labour within 2 weeks and 90% within 3 weeks. The risk of maternal coagulopathy is rare before 3–4 weeks has elapsed from the time of the IUD (with the exception of abruption) Br J Obstet Gynaecol 1997:4.

Causes

- Fetal causes: anomaly (including chromosomal), immune and non-immune hydrops fetalis, abruption and cord accidents.
- Maternal causes: pre-eclampsia and other medical disorders (renal, diabetes mellitus, infection, connective tissue disorders, impaired placental function).
- In at least 20% of cases no cause is found.

Check

- FBC and clotting.
- Kleihauer–Betke stain (? feto-maternal transfusion).
- HbA1C and random glucose.
- Lupus anticoagulant, anticardiolipin antibodies and thrombophilia screen (associated with impaired fetal outcome see p. 111).
- TORCH screen and parvovirus B_{19} for the presence of IgM, or a change in IgG from the booking sample.

If clinically there has been an abruption, see page 80. Otherwise, induce labour with mifepristone and misoprostol (Eur J Obstet Gynaecol 1996;70:159), but avoid membrane rupture until as late as possible as there is a very high chance of chorioamnionitis.

After-care

- Counselling.
- Offer of both religious support and time alone with the baby is essential.
- Also offer photos, handprints, a hair lock and help with the funeral arrangements.
- Discuss postmortem and chromosome studies.
- Give cabergoline 1 mg PO stat. to suppress lactation (side-effect: nausea).

- The parents are required to take a Stillbirth Certificate to the Registrar of Births and Deaths within 42 days.
- Discuss any local support group (e.g. SANDS)
- Arrange contraception (psychological problems are greater in those who become pregnant again within the first 6 months).
- Arrange a follow-up appointment (in about 4–6 weeks) to discuss the results.

MINOR DISORDERS OF PREGNANCY

Anaemia

Could there be a haemoglobinopathy? Check the ethnic origin and consider electrophoresis (p. 22). As there is a physiological fall in haemoglobin as pregnancy advances, there is controversy about the treatment of mild anaemia (e.g. Hb 8–10 g/dl). Iron supplements may lead to GI side-effects, have no proven benefits and carry theoretical worries about increasing the risks of 'sludging' within the placenta. On the other hand, iron supplements have no proven harmful effects, and may lead to improvements in mitochondrial function and generalized well-being. Most practitioners will prescribe oral $FeSO_4$ if the Hb is <10 g/dl or if the MCV is low (e.g. <80 fl), but it may be worth checking folate, vitamin B_{12} and ferritin before deciding on therapy. Oral iron is very well absorbed and the only indication for parenteral iron is when there are compliance worries or prohibitive side-effects with the oral route. Parenteral iron should never be given in thalassaemia.

Backache

This occurs as ligaments relax. Check for signs of nerve involvement. A support brace (e.g. Fembrace), a firm mattress and flat shoes help.

Carpal tunnel syndrome

The median nerve, which supplies the thumb, index and middle fingers, is compressed under the flexor retinaculum. Holding the wrist hyperflexed for 2 minutes reproduces the symptoms (this is more accurate than Tinel's test). Treatment is with splints, a local hydrocortisone injection or division of the retinaculum.

Constipation

This is common and usually responds to a high-fibre diet or laxatives. Avoid stimulant laxatives.

Cramps in the legs

This affects 33% of women in pregnancy and will be severe in 5%. Try elevating the end of the bed 20 cm. Salt is of unproven benefit and quinine should not be used.

Itching

This may be localized to the perineum or may be generalized. Localized itching may be due to infection (particularly candidiasis but, less commonly, pediculosis pubis or trichomonas vaginalis). Generalized itching may occur with eczema, urticaria or scabies. If there is a systemic rash, consider one of the four pregnancy-associated dermatoses (Table 2.3). Itching may also be due to intrahepatic cholestasis of pregnancy (see p. 125).

Nausea

See Hyperemesis, p. 46.

Oedema

This is very common in the ankle. Exclude pre-eclampsia and consider DVT. Elevation and support stockings are a help. Diuretics should not be used.

Reflux oesophagitis and heartburn

These occur secondary to relaxation of the oesophageal sphincter and pressure from the gravid uterus. Small meals should be taken often and cigarettes avoided. Antacids are helpful and there has been no reported teratogenicity with ranitidine.

TABLE 2.3 Dematoses of pregnancy

	Incidence	Features	Usual timing of onset	Fetal problems	Treatment
Pemphigoid gestationis	1:10 000	Pruritic erythematous papules, plaques and wheals spreading from the periumbilical area to the breasts, thighs and palms. Diagnosed by the presence of immunofluorescence of biopsy	9 weeks' gestation to 7 weeks postpartum	IUGR and increased fetal abnormality	Antihistamines, topical steroids, systemic steroids and, rarely, plasmapheresis
Polymorphic eruption of pregnancy	1:240	Urticaria and vesicles (with no bullae), rarely occurring in the periumbilical area	32 weeks' gestation to term	None	Antihistamines and topical steroids
Prurigo of pregnancy	1:300	Excoriated pustules on extensor surfaces	25–30 weeks' gestation	None	Antihistamines and topical steroids
Pruritic folliculitis		Acneiform rash	16–40 weeks' gestation	None	Topical steroids

Urinary frequency and stress incontinence

These usually resolve postnatally, but pelvic floor exercises can be commenced antenatally. Exclude a UTI.

MULTIPLE PREGNANCY

The UK incidence of twins is 12:1000 (3:1000 of these are monzygous). Worldwide the incidence ranges from 54:1000 in Nigeria to 4:1000 in Japan with the differences being almost entirely due to variations in dizygous rates. The incidence is higher with ovulation induction (e.g. with clomiphene 10%, with gonadotrophins 30%). The perinatal mortality in twin pregnancies is four or five times higher than for singleton pregnancies, largely related to preterm delivery (40% deliver before 37 weeks compared with 6% in singletons), IUGR, feto-fetal transfusion sequence (FFTS), malpresentation and an increased incidence of congenital malformations.

Chorionicity (i.e. number of placentae)

All dizygous pregnancies are dichorionic, and therefore have separate chorions and amnions. The placental tissue may appear to be continuous, but there are no significant vascular communications between the fetuses. Monozygotic pregnancies may also be dichorionic, but may be monochorionic diamniotic or monochorionic monoamniotic (Fig. 2.1). Most monochorionic placentas have interfetal vascular connections (Table 2.4).

TABLE 2.4 Chorionicity		
Chorionicity	Incidence (%)	Timing of separation (days)
Dichorionic, diamniotic	30	<4
Monochorionic, diamniotic	66	4–7
Monochorionic, monoamniotic	3	7–14
Conjoined twins	<1	Separation >14

Chorionicity determination is essential to allow risk stratification (Table 2.5), and has key implications for prenatal diagnosis and antenatal monitoring. It is most easily determined in the first or early second trimester:

- Widely separated first trimester sacs or separate placentae are dichorionic.
- Those with a 'lambda' or 'twin-peak' sign at the membrane insertion are dichorionic.
- Those with a dividing membrane >2 mm are often dichorionic.
- Different sex fetuses are always dichorionic (and dizygous).

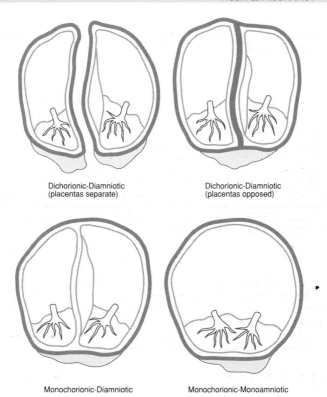

Dichorionic-Diamniotic
(placentas separate)

Dichorionic-Diamniotic
(placentas opposed)

Monochorionic-Diamniotic

Monochorionic-Monoamniotic

Fig. 2.1 Chorionicity in monzygotic pregnancies.

TABLE 2.5 Chorionicity and pregnancy outcome		
Outcome	Dichorionic (%)	Monochorionic (%)
Fetal loss before 24 weeks	1.8	2.2
Fetal loss after 24 weeks	1.6	2.8
Delivery before 32 weeks	5.5	9.2

The high early fetal mortality in monochorionic pregnancy before 24 weeks is probably largely due to severe early onset FFTS.

Fetal abnormality (Baillières Obstet Gynaecol 1998;12(1):19)
The incidence is no different per fetus in a dichorionic pregnancy compared
to a singleton pregnancy, but the incidence is greater with monochorionicity
(especially hydrocephalus, GI atresia and cardiac defects).

Structural defects These are usually confined to one twin (i.e. non-concordant),
e.g. if there is an NTD in one twin, the other twin is normal in 85–90%.
All multiple pregnancies should be offered a detailed midtrimester USS.
Selective termination with intracardiac KCl is possible in dichorionic
pregnancies only, and is most safely carried out before 16–20 weeks
(Am J Obstet Gynecol 1994:1265).

Chromosomal abnormalities These are usually discordant in dizygotic twins
and usually concordant in monozygotic twins. NT measurement is probably
more appropriate than serum screening for multiple pregnancies (but note
that NT may be slightly increased in normal monochorionic gestations).
Two amniocenteses are required in dichorionic pregnancies (very great care
must be taken to document which sample has come from which sac). CVS is
less appropriate for twin pregnancies, as it is difficult to be sure that both
placentas have been sampled, particularly if they are lying close together.

Management of pregnancy
At the initial visit:

- As many as 50% of twins diagnosed in the first trimester will proceed only
  as singletons despite the absence of PV loss. Parents should be told this if
  twins are diagnosed in the first trimester. Ensure chorionicity is established
  at the first scan. Consider starting $FeSO_4$ 200 mg/day and folate 5 mg/day.
- The parents are often quite shocked, so try and focus on the positive aspects
  while outlining that closer monitoring will be required. This can be
  expanded on later. Discuss whether antenatal screening should be
  performed, opening up to them the potential problems of finding one
  normal and one abnormal twin.

Thereafter, scan at:

- 18 weeks for growth discrepancy ±fetal abnormality if the patient wishes;
- 24 weeks for growth (the average weight for twins is 10% lighter than
  singletons);
- and 2–4 weekly thereafter for growth (more frequently if there is size
  discordance) ±Doppler, CTG and biophysical profile studies if appropriate.

Antenatal problems specific to multiple pregnancies

Feto-fetal transfusion sequence (FFTS) (Twin–twin transfusion syndrome)
This complicates 4–35% of monochorionic multiple pregnancies and accounts
for 15–17% of perinatal mortality in twins. The recipient develops severe

polyhydramnios with raised amniotic pressure, while the donor develops oliguria, oligohydramnios and growth restriction. This amniotic fluid discrepancy is used to establish the diagnosis and is supported by discordant growth measurements (although the inherent inaccuracy measurements of these makes them less useful diagnostic criteria). Contrary to previous thinking, the haemoglobin levels are often not discordant.

Most centres support serial amnioreductions if the AFI exceeds a certain limit or if the uterus becomes tense; it may be necessary to remove many thousands of millilitres over a number of occasions (RCOG Study Group 1995:56). Other centres support laser division of placental vessels (Br J Obstet Gynaecol 1998;446). There has been no randomized trial between the two techniques, but plans for such a trial are underway (www.eurofetus.org). More recently, it has been suggested that all that is required is a small disruption in the dividing membrane (Am J Obstet Gynecol 1997;176:S19).

Twins with one fetal death (RCOG Study Group 1995:218) First-trimester IUD in a twin has not been shown to have adverse consequences for the survivor. This probably also holds true for the early second trimester, but loss in the late second or third trimester commonly precipitates labour and 90% will have delivered within 3 weeks. Prognosis for a surviving dichorionic fetus is then influenced primarily by its gestation. When a monochorionic twin dies in utero, however, there are additional risks of death (approximately 20%) or cerebral damage (approximately 25%) in the co-twin. It is unlikely that immediate delivery will affect the risk of cerebral injury in the survivor.

Twin reversed arterial perfusion sequence (acardia) This is very rare and there is a high incidence of mortality in the donor twin due to intrauterine cardiac failure and prematurity. Cord ligation has been used in isolated cases.

MANAGEMENT OF TWIN DELIVERY

The commonest twin presentations are cephalic/cephalic (40%), cephalic/breech (40%), breech/cephalic (10%) and others, e.g. transverse (10%). Triplets and higher order multiples are probably best delivered by caesarean section. In general with twins, providing the first twin is cephalic, evidence would suggest that a trial of labour is appropriate. With significant growth discordance, particularly if the second twin is the smaller, it may be a reason to consider caesarean section. It is common practice to carry out a caesarean section at 38 weeks in those not suitable for a vaginal delivery, and to induce at 38–40 weeks those who are suitable but have not established labour spontaneously. If the labour is preterm (<34 weeks), many clinicians would also consider delivery by caesarean section.

Labour

Establish IV access and send blood for group and save. An epidural may be very useful in assisting the delivery of a second twin. The first stage is managed as for singleton pregnancies, except that the first twin is monitored with a fetal scalp electrode and the second twin is monitored abdominally. An experienced obstetrician, anaesthetist, two paediatricians and two midwives should be present for delivery, and a syntocinon infusion should be ready in case uterine activity falls away after delivery of the first twin (there is no literature on the rate of infusion, but starting at 3 mU/min increasing in 30 min to 6 mU/min is considered acceptable by many, see p. 68).

After delivery of the first twin it is often helpful to have someone 'stabilize' the second twin by abdominal palpation while a VE is performed to assess the station of the presenting part. If a second bag of membranes is present, it should not be broken until the presenting part has descended into the pelvis. If the second twin lies transverse after the delivery of the first twin, external cephalic or breech version is appropriate. If still transverse (particularly likely if the back is towards the fundus), the choice is between breech extraction (gentle continuous traction on one or both feet through intact membranes) or caesarean section. There is an increased incidence of PPH.

TRIPLETS AND HIGHER MULTIPLES

For those with higher order multiples, reduction to twins at 12–14 weeks may be considered (Baillières Obstet Gynecol 1998;12(1):147). With quadruplets or greater, there is likely to be overall benefit. For triplets, the situation is less clear. The miscarriage rate is increased (7.6% vs 2.6%) but the number delivering between 24 and 32 weeks is lower (8.2% vs 24.0%). Since severe preterm delivery is associated with risks of neonatal death and severe handicap, reduction to twins may not improve the chance of survival, but may reduce the rate of handicap. Whether these small benefits are justifiable on medical grounds alone, however, is difficult to assess, as a significant proportion of couples suffer long-term guilt.

Most clinicians would deliver those with triplets or higher order gestations by caesarean section because of problems with malpresentation and difficulties with intrapartum fetal monitoring.

PLACENTA PRAEVIA AND PAINLESS PV BLEEDING ANTENATALLY

(See also Haemorrhage, p. 80.)

There may be minimal or no PV loss in a large abruption and an abruption is usually, but not always, painful. There may be rapid and severe haemorrhage from a placenta praevia.

> **Remember**
>
> *Never* perform a VE in the presence of PV bleeding without first excluding a praevia. 'No PV until no PP.'

Placenta praevia

- Minor: — I   encroaches on lower segment,
        — II   (marginal) reaches internal os.
- Major: — III (partial) covers part of os,
        — IV (complete).

The incidence increases with maternal age and previous caesarean sections. Two per cent of those with a low-lying placenta before 24 weeks, 5% of those at 24–29 weeks and 23% of those at ≥30 weeks will still have a praevia at term. Symptomatic placenta praevias, and sometimes asymptomatic ones, are often managed on an inpatient basis if >30 weeks' gestation with elective delivery at 38 weeks' gestation. There is some evidence to support outpatient management of asymptomatic praevias, as well those symptomatic ones in which there has only been a small amount of bleeding (usually after a short inpatient stay).

Consider delivery of grade I vaginally (engagement of the presenting part is probably more important than the actual distance of placenta from os on USS). If there is doubt pre-induction or in early labour, an EUA may be of help. Placenta praevia sections should be supervised/performed by a senior obstetrician, and a large blood loss should be anticipated.

If the placenta invades the myometrium it is termed *placenta accreta*. If it reaches the serosa, it is termed *placenta increta*, and if through the serosa, it is termed *percreta*. The incidence of placenta accreta is higher after previous caesarean sections (see PPH, p. 81).

Painless PV spotting

This is common. Check the patient's history (pain, postcoital, date of last smear) and blood group. Confirm that the uterus is soft (contractions with labour, hard between contractions with abruption) and check for engagement (if engaged, it is not placenta praevia). Arrange a USS to check the placental site (even large abruptions may not be seen on USS) and, providing there is no praevia, using a speculum look for cervical effacement, dilatation, an ectropion and (only very rarely) carcinoma. If all is normal it is common practice to admit the patient until the bleeding settles. Many clinicians will not admit the patient if the bleeding is slight and is seen to be coming from an ectropion.

POLYHYDRAMNIOS

This may be defined as more than 2–3 litres of amniotic fluid, but for practical clinical purposes may be considered as:

- a single pool >8 cm,
- an amniotic fluid index >90th centile (Fig. 2.2).

It occurs in 0.5–2% of all pregnancies and is associated with maternal diabetes (≈20%) and congenital fetal anomaly (≈5%), particularly:

- Obstruction: oesophageal atresia (commonly in tracheo-oesophageal fistula), duodenal atresia (see p. 19), small intestine or colonic obstruction (atresia, Hirschsprung's disease, see p. 30).
- High urine output: macrosomia, recipient of twin–twin transfusion (see p. 52), or placental or fetal tumour.
- Neuromuscular poor swallowing (rare): anencephaly, myotonic dystrophy (see p. 31), maternal myaesthenia, fetal akinesia sequence or spinal muscular atrophy.
- Mechanical (very rare): facial tumour, macroglossia or micrognathia.

Even in the absence of an identifiable cause (>60%), polyhydramnios is associated with an increased rate of caesarean section, antepartum fetal death (0.6% vs 0.2%), postpartum death (2.8% vs 0.4%), abruption (0.9% vs 0.3%), malpresentation (6.8% vs 2.9%), cord prolapse (2.2% vs 0.3%) and carrying a large for gestational age infant (24% vs 8%). (Eur J Obstet Gynaecol Reprod Biol 1998;77:157).

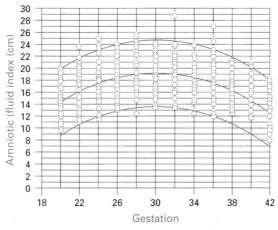

Fig. 2.2 Gestation reference range (mean ± 2 SD) for amniotic fluid index (Br J Obstet Gynaecol 1993:531).

Investigations

USS (fetal anomaly scan, growth and skeletal survey), GTT, Rhesus status and fetal well-being assessment.

Management

- Conservative management is ideal, but options include:
  — tapping (may lead to infection or preterm labour), *PROM , abruption*
  — indomethacin 25 g QID PO decreases fetal urine production, but carries the risk of ductus arteriosis constriction or irreversible fetal renal impairment.
- Increased antenatal fetal surveillance.
- Awareness of the risks of intrapartum complications.
- Paediatric involvement at delivery.

Sulindac 100mg BD ↓ Less effect on ductus & Kidney

PRELABOUR RUPTURE OF MEMBRANES (PROM)

> Occurs in 6–12% of live births.

TERM

- In 70% of cases rupture of membranes is established in labour by 24 hours and in 90% by 48 hours. Providing, therefore, that the mother is apyrexial, the baby is in cephalic presentation, the liquor is clear and the CTG is normal a case may be made for adopting a conservative policy for 48 hours (Br J Obstet Gynaecol 1996:755). There is also evidence, however, that induction of labour on admission may reduce the incidence of neonatal infection with no increase in caesarean section (N Engl J Med 1996:1005). Delivery must be undertaken at once (ideally by caesarean section unless labour is well established) if there is a clinical suspicion of chorioamnionitis with pyrexia or meconium (pain and discharge are late features).
- Accurate diagnosis is vital. Speculum examination is not essential if the diagnosis is obvious, but may be used to take an HVS and to establish the diagnosis by presence of liquor with vernix, meconium or ferning.

 A digital vaginal examination is not indicated if the mother is not in labour.

PRETERM (<37 weeks)

- Occurs in 2–3% of all pregnancies but in 40–60% of all pre-term deliveries. It is associated with polyhydramnios, twins and infection (especially group B streptococcus, gonococcus, mycoplasma and, rarely, listeria). Up to a third may occur secondary to infection.
- Scan to confirm presentation. The biophysical profile is difficult to interpret without the parameter of liquor volume. Absence of fetal breathing movements *may* indicate infection, but prolonged scanning (>30 min) may be required.
- Check the temperature, an MSU and the WCC (rises after maternal steroids) ± c-reactive protein (a better predictor of chorioamnionitis, but still with low sensitivity).
- It may be considered appropriate to carry out a sterile speculum examination to take an HVS and to establish the diagnosis (see above), but an HVS is not a predictor of subsequent infection and such procedures may themselves introduce infection.

> ⚠ **A digital vaginal examination is not indicated if the mother is not in labour.**

Management of preterm prelabour rupture of membranes (PPROM)

- Give dexamethasone or betamethasone 24 mg IM over 48 hours if <34 weeks. There is currently no consensus regarding repeating courses of corticosteroids if the patient remains undelivered >7 days after the original course.
- Routine antibiotics (e.g. ampicillin 1 g PO/IV QID or erythromycin 500 mg PO QD) increases the number of women undelivered at 7 days and reduces neonatal and maternal morbidity. Antibiotics have not been shown to improve neonatal survival (Lancet 1995;346:1271), but do prolong gestational age. Many consider it appropriate to start antibiotics in all cases. *ORACLE*
- Most mothers will establish in labour (e.g. ≈75% at 28 weeks establish within 7 days). Do not give tocolytics unless contracting and you are certain that there is no chorioamnionitis. There is no evidence that tocolysis is beneficial in the presence of PPROM, and the use of tocolytics can only be justified in highly selected cases.
- Regular fetal monitoring is essential.
- If the mother does not establish in labour, the problem is one of balancing the risks of chorioamnionitis (which accounts for 20% of neonatal deaths) against the risks of delivery. Infection supervenes after membranes have

ruptured in 0.5% and 25% of cases, depending on the criteria employed for diagnosis. The incidence increases with the number of VEs performed.

- It is considered acceptable practice to manage these patients on an outpatient basis following an initial inpatient stay, the patient may take her own temperature at home on a QID basis. It is also common practice to deliver if >36 weeks.
- If infection develops, take blood cultures and give antibiotics (e.g. ampicillin 500 mg IV QID and gentamicin – see dosage p. 104). Deliver ASAP, ideally by caesarean section, unless labour is well established.
- The outcome becomes more guarded the earlier membrane rupture occurs on account of pulmonary hypoplasia and severe skeletal deformities (see p. 24). Pulmonary hypoplasia occurs in 50% with SRM before 20 weeks and 3% after 24 weeks. Lung size, amniotic fluid volume and fetal breathing movements on antenatal ultrasound are not reliable predictors of pulmonary hypoplasia.

PROLONGED PREGNANCY (>42 weeks)

1:1000 @ 37wks / 3:1000 @ 42wk / 6:1000 @ 43 wk

> This occurs in 10% of pregnancies and is associated with an increased perinatal mortality (perinatal mortality is 5:1000 between 37 and 42 weeks and 9.7:1000 after 42 weeks) due to IUD, intrapartum hypoxia and meconium aspiration syndrome. Dating the pregnancy by ultrasound before 18 weeks is more reliable than LMP in reducing the incidence of prolonged pregnancy. *

Sweeping the membranes If this is done once after 40 weeks it doubles the incidence of spontaneous labour over controls, especially in those with a low Bishop's score. The risk of infection is considered to be minimal (Br J Obstet Gynaecol 1993:889). The procedure is uncomfortable.

Induction of labour At >41 weeks this reduces the incidence of fetal distress and meconium staining over those managed conservatively with monitoring (N Engl J Med 1992:1587). There is also a reduction in the caesarean section rate and no increase in the incidence of uterine hypertonus. No demonstrable effect on perinatal mortality has been demonstrated. It has been estimated, however, that 500 inductions may be required to prevent one perinatal death. Dissatisfaction of labour is strongly associated with operative delivery, and is not associated with induction of labour (Br J Obstet Gynaecol 1986:1059).

Monitoring of postdates pregnancy The use of ultrasound and CTG confers no demonstrable benefit, but is frequently performed.

SMALL FETUS (SGA and IUGR)

> Small for gestational age (SGA) refers to those fetuses that weigh <10th centile for gestational age. They may simply be inherently small, but healthy and growing along their centile. Intrauterine growth retardation (IUGR) refers to any fetus failing to achieve its growth potential. Not all small-for-dates (SFD) fetuses are growth retarded, and not all growth-retarded fetuses are SFD.

The small fetus carries an increased risk of intrauterine death, intrapartum asphyxia, neonatal hypoglycaemia and possible long-term neurological impairment. The perinatal mortality is also higher:

- >10th centile overall, 12:1000;
- 5th–10th centile, 22:1000;
- <5th centile, 190:1000 (80% occur in utero, with 50% of these occurring after 36 weeks).

In theory, a SGA fetus that has a normal growth velocity is likely to be simply inherently small, whereas a baby with IUGR (i.e. reduced growth velocity) should be investigated further. In reality, the two are often initially managed in the same way, as the difference only becomes apparent with time. Risk factors for IUGR include smoking, previous SGA babies and 'unexplained' increased αFP.

Causes of IUGR

- Uteroplacental insufficiency: pre-eclampsia, abruption or unexplained.
- Fetal factors: congenital abnormality (17% in those <5th centile), congenital infection or in association with multiple pregnancy.
- Maternal factors: smoking, nutrition, alcohol, drugs, Rhesus iso-immunization or medical problems (severe anaemia, or cardiovascular, renal or GI pathology).

Diagnosis

This follows antenatal screening. Clinical examination has a 40–50% sensitivity and USS a 25–90% sensitivity. The specificity of USS is better. The use of computer-generated customized growth charts improves the identification of IUGR (Br J Obstet Gynaecol 1998:531).

Management

- History for the above maternal causes.
- BP and urine dipsticks to exclude pre-eclampsia.
- USS for fetal anomaly.

- Vascular resistance assessment with Doppler studies, and fetal well-being assessment with biophysical profile and CTG (see Liquor Volume, Fig. 2.2).
- It is usually impossible to minimize causal factors (except smoking).
- Steroids should be given if delivery before 34 weeks is anticipated (see p. 70).

The frequency of monitoring in the non-compromised fetus depends on many factors, but it may be possible to monitor on an outpatient basis every 1–14 days. Inpatient monitoring or delivery should be considered if the fetus is compromised. Decisions about the timing and mode of delivery are often difficult and depend on all of the above factors (see also Fetal Monitoring, p. 74).

ACUTE OBSTETRICS

OBSTETRICAL PROBLEMS

NORMAL LABOUR

> Normal labour begins spontaneously at 37–42 weeks, progresses at an acceptable rate (see below) and results in the spontaneous vaginal delivery of a live undistressed neonate in the occipitoanterior position.

The first stage is from the onset of labour until full dilatation of the cervix. Onset may be, but does not need to be, preceded by a show (mucus or small amount of blood-stained discharge), and true labour is said to have begun when there is both regular uterine activity and cervical dilatation. There may be an initial and sometimes prolonged (hours or days) latent phase before true labour begins, but an acceptable rate of dilatation after 3 cm is 1 cm/h in a primigravida and 1–2 cm/h in a multigravida. SRM may occur prior to the onset of labour (see p. 57), but more usually some time after contractions have started. The head usually engages at the pelvic brim in the occipitotransverse position (see Fig. 3.2a), flexing as it descends into the pelvic cavity and rotating to occipitoanterior at the level of the ischial spines. Progress should be charted on a partogram (Fig. 3.1) together with maternal pulse, blood pressure, temperature, fetal heart rate, cervical dilatation, descent of the presenting part, frequency of contractions and presence or absence of meconium. It is reasonable to carry out a vaginal examination at least every 4 hours to assess dilatation, descent (relative to ischial spines), position, caput and moulding (≥1 if the sutures are aligned, ≥2 if overlapping, ≥3 if irreducible). In low-risk mothers the fetal heart rate may be monitored either intermittently (approximately every 15 minutes, with a reading taken before, during and after a contraction) or continuously with a cardiotocograph (see p. 74).

The second stage is from full dilatation until delivery of the baby (Fig. 3.2 b–e). There may be an initial passive (non-pushing) phase before the desire to push is felt, followed by an active (pushing) stage. The head extends as it descends, distending the vulva until it is delivered. It then externally rotates to the transverse position again as the shoulders are rotated within the pelvis to the AP plane and the anterior shoulder is delivered by downward lateral traction of the trunk, with subsequent upward lateral traction being used for the posterior shoulder. The rest of the baby usually follows without difficulty. Normal time for the second stage is 1–3 hours in a primigravida and 1 hour or less in a multigravida.

This third stage is from delivery of the baby until delivery of the placenta. The uterus contracts, shearing the placenta from the uterine wall; this separation is often indicated by a small rush of dark blood and a lengthening of cord. The placenta can then be delivered by gentle cord traction (see Retained

START PARTOGRAM AT CERVICAL DILATION AT FIRST VE PLOTTED ONTO APPROPRIATE POINT ON LINE

TIME PARTOGRAM STARTED

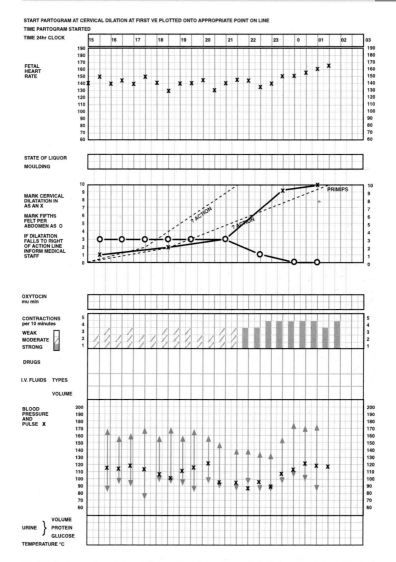

Fig. 3.1 Partogram for primigravid labour. The partogram graph for parous labour is steeper (see text).

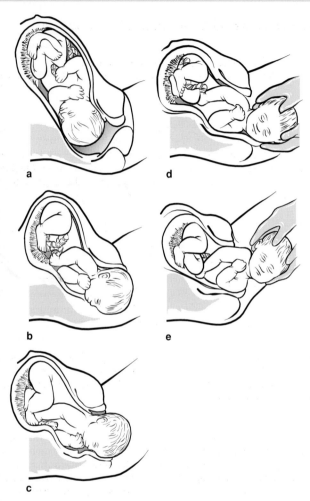

Fig. 3.2 **a** Full dilatation. **b** Descent of the head with extension and rotation of the head. **c** The shoulders remain behind the symphysis pubis. **d** External rotation of the head and delivery of the anterior shoulder. **e** Delivery of the posterior shoulder.

Placenta), but caution is required to avoid uterine inversion (see p. 94). The routine use of Syntocinon 10 IU IM following delivery of the anterior shoulder reduces the risk of PPH by about 60% (no significant difference in effectiveness to syntometrine, with a lower incidence of vomiting).

INDUCTION AND AUGMENTATION OF LABOUR

> Induction of labour refers only to a mother not in labour.
> Augmentation is the process of accelerating progress after labour has begun.

Induction

The main risks are of inappropriate use, hyperstimulation and failed induction. Review the gestation, indication and presentation, and assess the cervix using the modified Bishop's Scoring System (Table 3.1). Caution is required with previous caesarean section, previous precipitate labour, or if highly parous. Monitor with CTG at least before induction and as soon as there is uterine activity.

TABLE 3.1 Bishop's Scoring System for cervical assessment				
Score	**0**	**1**	**2**	**3**
Cervical dilatation (cm)	<1	1–2	2–4	>4
Length of cervix (cm)	>4	2–4	1–2	<1
Station of presenting part (cm)	Spines −3	Spines −2	Spines −1	At or below spines
Consistency	Firm	Average	Soft	
Position	Posterior	Central	Anterior	

- If the score is <7, 'ripen' the cervix with prostaglandins (gel or pessary).
- If the score is >6, consider either prostaglandins or ARM ± Syntocinon (there may be greater patient satisfaction with the former, but the latter may allow more control).

Prostaglandins

Intravaginal prostaglandin E_2 (PGE$_2$) gel has fewer side-effects than oral preparations and also has a lower failure rate than using the intracervical route. The gel (e.g. Prostin) is inserted into the posterior fornix. Give primigravidae 2 mg gel and multiparae 1 mg gel. If there is no uterine activity, reassess in 6 hours. If the Bishop's score is <7, give a further 1 mg and reassess again 6 hours later. Further doses may then be given, or the patient may be left for 12–18 hours (e.g. overnight). The maximum quoted dose is 4 mg in primigravidae and 3 mg in multiparae, but some practitioners consider it appropriate to give more than this. If at any stage the Bishop's score is >6, perform an ARM, reassess in a further 2 hours and start Syntocinon if there is still no change. Gel should not be given if there is uterine activity.

Sustained-release preparations are also available. Propess is a polymer-based vaginal insert with retrieval thread containing 10 mg PGE$_2$. It is placed in the posterior fornix for 12 hours (only 5 mg prostaglandin is released over this time), after which it is removed. This technique has the advantage that the pessary can be removed if hyperstimulation develops, and trials indicate that it is probably safe. It has not been shown to be superior to gel.

Artificial rupture of membranes (ARM)

ARM (amniotomy) is used to induce labour in those with a sufficiently favourable cervix and is also used for augmentation (see below). Further, it allows assessment of the colour of the liquor (see Meconium, p. 78). Its routine use in early labour is surrounded by a degree of controversy, as it can be argued that there is less cushioning of the fetal head and therefore a greater incidence of fetal heart rate decelerations (see p. 76). Early ARM and Syntocinon probably do not confer benefit over conservative management in nulliparous women with mild delays in early spontaneous labour (Br J Obstet Gynaecol 1998:189).

The fetal head should be well applied to the cervix to minimize the risk of cord prolapse. With asepsis, the tips of the index and middle fingers of one hand should be placed through the cervix onto the membranes (Fig. 3.3). The amni-hook should be allowed to slide down the groove between these fingers (the hook pointing downwards towards the fingers) until the cervix is reached. The point is then turned upwards to break the membrane sac. Liquor is usually seen, but may be absent in oligohydramnios or with a well-engaged head. Exclude cord prolapse before removing fingers. Check the FH. Absent liquor following ARM should be treated as meconium staining until proven otherwise (see p. 78).

Syntocinon

This may be used for induction following ARM with a favourable cervix, or for augmentation of a slow, non-obstructed labour. It should only be started if the membranes have been ruptured, and continuous CTG monitoring is mandatory. Make up a 500 ml infusion of 0.9% saline (or Hartmann's

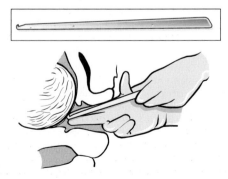

Fig. 3.3 Artificial rupture of the membranes (ARM).

solution) with 10 U of Syntocinon. The dose should be titrated against the contractions, aiming for not more than 6–7 every 15 minutes. Start at 3 ml/h (1 mU/min), increasing every 30 minutes by 3 ml/h until at 12 ml/h. Then increase by 6 ml/h every 30 min to 36 ml/h (12 mU/min) (Br J Obstet Gynaecol 1993:786). This regimen may be halved in highly parous women (>5 labours).

For induction, the use of Syntocinon immediately following ARM reduces the time to delivery, the rates of PPH and the need for operative delivery. As labour will begin within 24 hours in 88% of cases, however, it is unclear whether these advantages outweigh the maternal inconvenience of an IV infusion, restricted mobility and continuous fetal monitoring. An individual approach is advised.

Augmentation

The cause of failure to progress must be considered carefully.

- Obstruction may be caused by the baby being too big or the pelvis too small (true cephalopelvic disproportion) or by malposition (relative cephalopelvic disproportion). There may be a clinical suspicion from abdominal palpation, and there is likely to be caput or moulding at VE.
- Inadequate dilatation may also be due to inadequate contractions. 'Adequacy' of contractions is very difficult to assess, and some degree of judgement rests with experience and the absence of any evidence of obstruction. If there is felt to be true poor uterine activity it is reasonable to start Syntocinon cautiously, as above.

PRETERM LABOUR (if appropriate, see Prelabour Rupture of Membranes, p. 57)

> This is defined as labour occurring at 24–37 weeks. It occurs in 6–10% of pregnancies, and in about 30% of cases is due to direct medical intervention. Although it may be associated with multiple pregnancy, APH, IUGR, cervical incompetence, amnionitis, congenital uterine anomaly, polyhydramnios or systemic infection, particularly pyelonephritis, many cases are 'idiopathic'.

There have been a number of techniques proposed to screen for preterm labour. A cervical length of <15 mm at 23 weeks (measured by TV USS) occurs in 2% of the population but accounts for 90% and 60% of those who will deliver at ≤28 and ≤32 weeks, respectively. The risk of preterm labour with a cervical length of 15 mm is 4%, rising to 78% at a length of <5 mm. The value of this knowledge is unclear as it remains unknown, for example, whether a cervical suture is indicated, is of no help, or is even contraindicated in such circumstances. The presence of fetal fibronectin measured at 23 weeks (a connective tissue protein in fetal membranes) predicts 60% of spontaneous preterm births at <28 weeks in an unselected population, although with a PPV of only 25% (Obstet Gynecol 1996;87:643). In those suspected to be in preterm labour, a positive test has a PPV of 77%, and <3% of mothers with a negative test will deliver in the next 3 weeks (Br J Obstet Gynecol 1996;103:648). Benefit from screening for any of the above has not been shown.

Screening for infection has also been considered, but again no benefits have been demonstrated. Bacterial vaginosis, which is present in 10–20% of pregnant women, has been associated with a twofold relative risk of preterm delivery. There is probably reasonable evidence to support treating such an infection in high-risk groups (Am J Obstet Gynecol 1997;177:375). For group B β-haemolytic streptococci, see page 137).

Assessment and management

- Is preterm labour likely? Are there palpable contractions (you may need to sit and palpate the uterus)? Is the cervix closed (avoid VE if SRM)?
- Assess fetal and maternal state. Is there evidence of maternal haemorrhage or pyrexia? Is there cephalic presentation of the fetus? Is an FH present? CTG if >approx. 28 weeks?
- Alert paediatricians. Could they cope with this baby? Arrange in utero transfer if necessary.
- Give steroids. These should be given if delivery before 34 weeks is likely. Use betamethasone or dexamethasone 24 mg IM in divided doses over 24 hours. This significantly reduces the incidence of respiratory distress syndrome (by ≈50%), necrotizing enterocolitis and periventricular haemorrhage. There is debate about steroid use in those 34–37 weeks pregnant, but note that 94 women in this group will need to be treated to prevent 1 case of RDS (compared with 5:1 at 31 weeks). No adverse neurological or cognitive effects following steroid treatment have been demonstrated in those followed for up to 12 years, but the possibility of unrecognized long-term effects has not been excluded. There is no identifiable increase in the incidence of maternal or fetal infection, but steroids are contraindicated with active maternal septicaemia/TB. It is unknown whether it is appropriate to prescribe repeat doses (e.g 12 mg every 10 days) if delivery risk is still present. It is hoped that the TEAM (Trial of the Effects of Antenatal Multiple Courses of Steroids versus a Single Course) study will provide this answer. Great caution should be used in IDDM as steroids lead to secondary hyperglycaemia and possible DKA (IV control with insulin and dextrose may be appropriate).
- Consider antibiotics. It is postulated that preterm labour may in part be related to subclinical infection, and a broad-spectrum antibiotic may be appropriate. A large trial using combinations of augmentin 375 mg QID, erythromycin 250 mg QID and placebo is currently underway to assess whether antibiotic treatment might be helpful in reducing the incidence of delivery in threatened preterm labour (ORACLE trial).

- Consider tocolytics.
  - **Ritodrine** (Yutopar) **IV** has been shown to reduce the proportion of deliveries within the first 48 hours, although it has not been shown to be of benefit in terms of improved fetal morbidity or mortality. In view of the potentially serious maternal side-effects, its use should be restricted to those of <34 weeks' gestation undergoing in utero transfer to an appropriate neonatal unit and possibly for the purpose of steroid administration. *There have been a number of maternal deaths associated with ritodrine (particularly when also used with steroids), and it must be used under close direct supervision.* It is contraindicated with maternal cardiac disease, hyperthyroidism, APH, severe pre-eclampsia and any other situation in which prolongation of pregnancy would be hazardous. The side-effects include maternal and fetal tachycardia (keep maternal P < 140 bpm) and pulmonary oedema. Rarely, severe maternal bradycardia, hypotension and arrhythmias may occur (especially SVT, AF and premature ventricular contractions) as well as visual disturbances, skin flushing, nausea, vomiting, hyperkalaemia and hyperglycaemia (therefore caution with IDDM and potassium sparing diuretics). Monitor the P and BP frequently (e.g. every 15 min), glucose and U&E (e.g. 4 hourly). Keep an accurate fluid balance and auscultate the bases (e.g. 4 hourly).
    - Ritodrine is supplied in ampoules (50 mg in 5 ml). For an infusion, add three ampoules (i.e. 15 ml, 150 mg drug) to 35 ml of 5% dextrose in a 50 ml syringe (1 ml/h = 50 μg/min). Start infusing at 1 ml/h, increasing by 1 ml/h every 15 min to a maximum of 7 ml/h (350 μg/min). When contractions stop (or if the maternal pulse is >140 bpm) reduce by 1 ml/h every 30 min.
    - If pulmonary oedema develops, stop the infusion, give O_2, sit the patient up, give frusemide 50 mg IV and morphine 10 mg IV. If there is an arrhythmia, stop the infusion, and check the potassium level.
  - **Nifedipine** (30 mg PO BD followed by 20 mg PO 8 hourly) may be effective and is safer than ritodrine.
  - **Indomethacin** (100 mg suppository OD PR). Trials have shown that this drug reduces the frequency of delivery within 48 hours and within 7–10 days from the beginning of treatment. It may lead to maternal GI irritation, peptic ulceration, thrombocytopenia, allergic reactions, headaches and dizziness. There are reports about partial closure of the fetal ductus arteriosis, impaired fetal renal function, bronchopulmonary dysplasia and persistent pulmonary hypertension in the neonatal period.

Cervical cerclage

Elective transvaginal cervical cerclage is probably of benefit in those with a history of cervical incompetence, particularly those with a history of more than two deliveries before 37 weeks (Br J Obstet Gynaecol 1993:516). In the quoted trial, there was benefit in only 1:25 of the relatively low-risk population.

Transabdominal cervicoisthmic cerclage is a specialist procedure reserved for failed transcervical cerclage.

'Rescue' cerclage refers to the emergency use of a suture in early preterm labour thought to be due to cervical incompetence, and may be used following the reduction of prolapsed membranes.

PRECIPITATE LABOUR

This occurs especially with induction of labour, augmentation and grand multiparity.

Management

- Stop Syntocinon if an infusion is running.
- Assess the fetal condition:
  — if there is acute 'distress', perform a VE and consider if vaginal delivery is possible;
  — if a caesarean section is considered, re-examine the patient in theatre immediately prior to starting (vaginal delivery may be possible).
- Hypertonus may respond to IV ritodrine (Yutopar). This is supplied in ampoules (50 mg in 5 ml). It is contraindicated with maternal cardiac disease and hyperthyroidism. The side-effects include maternal and fetal tachycardia (keep the maternal pulse <140 bpm) and pulmonary oedema. Rarely, severe maternal bradycardia, hypotension and arrhythmias may occur (especially SVT, AF and premature ventricular contractions) as well as visual disturbances, skin flushing, nausea, vomiting, hyperkalaemia and hyperglycaemia (therefore caution should be taken with IDDM and potassium sparing diuretics). Give the drug as follows:
  — Bolus: take 1 ml (i.e. 10 mg) and make up to 10 ml with normal saline. Give 1–3 ml of this solution (i.e. 1–3 mg) IV stat.
  — Then start an infusion. Add 3 ampoules (i.e. 150 mg) to 35 ml of 5% dextrose in a 50 ml syringe (therefore 1 ml = 50 µg/min). Start infusing at 1 ml/h, increasing by 1 ml/h every 10 min to a maximum of 7 ml/h (350 µg/min).
  — If pulmonary oedema develops, stop the infusion, give O_2, sit the patient up, give frusemide 50 mg IV and morphine 10 mg IV. If there is an arrhythmia, stop the infusion, and check the potassium level.

ANALGESIA FOR LABOUR

Antenatal relaxation training may engender calm, thus conserving energy. False expectations may induce distrust.

Psychological methods Randomized trials confirm that good support by a trained care-giver can reduce analgesia requirements. Although unsupported by trials, warm-water massage, transcutaneous electrical nerve stimulation (TENS), acupuncture, aromatherapy and reflexology are favoured by some.

Systemic opioid analgesia Pethidine 50–150 mg IM is favoured by many and, although it does not reduce the pain score in labour, many women feel that they mind the pain less. Some women feel disorientated and experience loss of control. Babies may require naloxone immediately postnatally. Diamorphine 5–10 mg IM is popular in a few centres, particularly in Scotland. It is good practice to prescribe an antiemetic at the same time.

Inhalational analgesia Entonox is a 50% nitrous oxide 50% oxygen mixture. It is probably more effective overall than Pethidine, although has little effect on pain score and may make women light-headed and nauseated.

Regional analgesia This is particularly valuable for prolonged or complicated labour (including twins) and for caesarean sections or instrumental delivery. Anaesthetic experience is essential:

- *Epidural*. A cannula is placed in the extradural space for repeated or continuous infusion of local anaesthetic, blocking the spinal nerves from the uterus and birth canal (T10–L1). It is the only form of labour analgesia to produce consistent reduction in the pain score, but it has potential problems:
  — Maternal problems: occasional failure to establish a block (total or partial); total spinal block; inadvertent spinal block; epidural haematomas.
  — Fetal problems: hypotension, leading to fetal compromise.
- *Spinal analgesia* (a single injection of local anaesthetic into the sub-arachnoid space) provides a dense block for 2–4 hours which is particularly useful for caesarean section or some instrumental deliveries.

Regional analgesia is contraindicated with a bleeding diathesis (including full anticoagulation), infection or hypovolaemia. It is likely to reduce the second stage desire to push, and may increase the need for instrumental delivery.

 If hypotension occurs secondary to distal vasodilation, ensure that the patient is on her side (or at least has 45° of lateral tilt) and give O₂. Take a 30 mg ampoule of ephedrine (1 ml) and dilute to 10 ml with normal saline (i.e. 3 mg/ml). Give 1 ml IV stat. and titrate the dose thereafter according to the response. There may be rebound hypertension.

FETAL MONITORING

> Always consider the background of previous fetal monitoring, gestation, growth, meconium and rate of progress in labour. If there is acute fetal distress, stop any Syntocinon, turn the mother onto her side, give O_2 and check the BP. If hyperstimulated, see p. 72.
>
> (For more detailed CTG interpretation see: Barea, Smith 1992 The CTG in practice, Churchill Livingstone).

Intermittent monitoring

Assessment of the fetal heart rate can be used to provide some information about fetal well-being. In 'low-risk' labours (see below), providing an admission CTG is normal, it is probably safe to auscultate the fetal heart every 15 minutes before and after a contraction, repeating a 20 minute CTG every 2–3 hours or if there are decelerations or a change in baseline rate on auscultation. A baseline tachycardia or bradycardia, or late decelerations (i.e. occurring after a contraction) are indications for further evaluation, often continuous CTG monitoring ±FBS ±intervention. The routine use of continuous CTG monitoring in low-risk labours may increase the rate of intervention for no demonstrable fetal benefit.

Continuous heart rate monitoring (CTG) (Fig. 3.4)

> A cardiotocograph measures fetal heart rate together with the timing of contractions. All those with risk factors (including IUGR, meconium, Syntocinon, epidurals and previous caesarean sections) should have continuous CTG monitoring. Check that you are looking at the correct patient's trace and that the paper speed is correct (1 cm/min). Intrapartum CTGs are usually used to screen those who may need further assessment (e.g. FBS ± intervention).

CTG with abdominal (Doppler) probe
Use DARTH VADER for thorough CTG evaluation:

D details (name, time, etc.)	**V** variability
A assess quality	**A** accelerations
R recorded fetal movements	**D** decelerations
T tocograph	**E** evaluation
H heart rate	**R** response

Heartrate baseline 110–160 bpm Tachycardia is associated with prematurity, fetal acidosis, maternal pyrexia, and the use of β-sympathomimetics. Baseline bradycardia is rarely associated with fetal acidosis (unless severe, e.g.

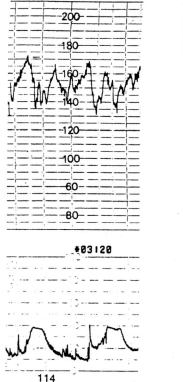

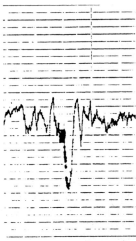

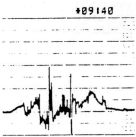

Fig. 3.4 a There is good variability, but the baseline is difficult to determine.

Fig. 3.4 b There is an early deceleration on the background of a 140 bpm baseline, with good variability and shouldering.

abruption or uterine rupture) and is more commonly found with maturity, hypotension, sedation and, rarely, congenital heart block. Cardiac dysrhythmias are rare but can cause extremes of heart rate, either fast or slow, with tachycardia being the more sinister.

Variability This gives the best indication of well-being, normal variability being 10–25 bpm. The commonest reason for loss of baseline variability is the 'sleep' or 'quiet' phase of the fetal behavioural cycle, which may last up to 40 minutes. Loss of variability is also associated with prematurity, acidosis and drugs (e.g. opiates or benzodiazepines). Reduced variability in the presence of late decelerations markedly increases the likelihood of fetal acidosis.

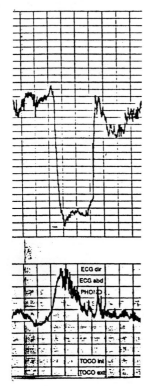

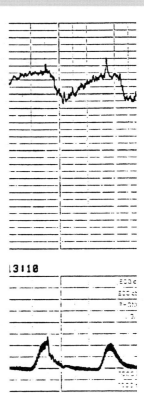

Fig. 3.4 c There is good variability with a 140–150 bpm baseline, and broad deep variable, possibly late, decelerations.

Fig. 3.4 d The baseline is 170–180 bpm, with reduced variability and shallow late decelerations. The features are highly suggestive of fetal distress.

Accelerations Remember the *'rule of 15'* for antenatal assessment: i.e. there should be at least two accelerations per 15 minutes with an amplitude greater than 15 bpm lasting for at least 15 seconds. There may be fewer accelerations in established labour.

Decelerations These are of at least 15 bpm and last for more than 15 seconds. Early decelerations occur with contractions. If they occur more than 15 seconds after the contraction they are termed 'late'. 'Variable' contractions vary in both timing and shape.

● *Early decelerations* reflect increased vagal tone (intracranial pressure rises during a contraction) and are physiological.

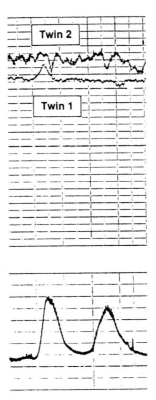

Fig. 3.4 e Some CTG monitors will add 20 bpm to the baseline of one twin to differentiate it from the other trace. There is reduced variability in twin 1, and the apparent acceleration does not fulfil the criteria for a true acceleration of 15 bpm.

- *Variable decelerations* may represent cord compression (e.g. in oligohydramnios) or acidosis. A small acceleration at the beginning and end of a deceleration (shouldering) suggest that the fetus is coping well with cord compression.
- *Late decelerations* suggest acidosis. Shallow late decelerations may be particularly ominous.

A true sinusoidal trace is rare. There is a smooth undulating sine-wave-like baseline with no variability. It may represent anaemia (especially with an amplitude >20 bpm at 1–2 oscillations/min) but can be a feature of fetal physiological behaviour. It should be considered to be serious until proven otherwise.

CTG with scalp clip (Fig. 3.5)

These are used to improve the quality of CTG traces if there is poor abdominal pick-up, or for monitoring the presenting fetus in multiple pregnancy. Their use is contraindicated where there may be a risk of vertical infection (HIV, HBV, HSV, etc.), a fetal bleeding diathesis (see p. 145) and in severe prematurity (e.g. <32–34 weeks).

Liquor assessment

> Meconium staining of the liquor is associated with an increased chance of fetal distress. A normal CTG provides reassurance, but an abnormal CTG becomes even more significant if meconium is present, and should lower the threshold for investigation or intervention.

As well as being a sign of fetal distress, meconium is found below the cords postnatally in about one-third of cases in which it is present, and may give rise to the meconium aspiration syndrome. Clinical features range from mild neonatal tachypnoea to severe respiratory compromise. The incidence is probably unrelated to pH (and indeed the majority of babies with meconium aspiration syndrome are not acidotic at delivery), but the syndrome is more likely to be severe if there is associated acidosis. It is also more severe when the meconium is thick. There is no evidence to support early delivery as a

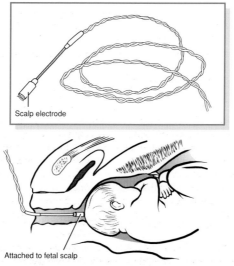

Scalp electrode

Attached to fetal scalp

Fig. 3.5 Fetal scalp electrode.

prophylactic measure in the absence of fetal distress, as it is likely that the aspiration occurs in utero rather than at delivery itself. It is therefore accepted by many that routine suction on the perineum carries no benefit (and may cause apnoeas and bradycardias). There is now some evidence from work in Africa supporting early intrapartum amnioinfusion to reduce the incidence of meconium aspiration syndrome (Br J Obstet Gynaecol 1998:304, 309). Normal saline (800 ml) is infused at 15 ml/min through a transcervical intrauterine catheter, and infusion is then maintained at 3 ml/min for the duration of labour. This is not standard UK practice at present.

Fetal pH measurement

Fetal blood sampling is almost always used to establish further information following a suspicious CTG and perhaps to prevent unnecessary intervention. Consider alternatives. For example, if the head is well down at full dilatation, delivery might be more appropriate, as it would also be if the cervix is insufficiently dilated and the CTG is clearly highly suspicious (e.g. preterminal bradycardia). A pH of >7.25 is normal, one of 7.20–7.25 is borderline and an abnormal pH is <7.20.

Association between CTG and pH (Obstet Gynecol 1975:392)

- If all 4 components of the CTG are normal, the risk of a pH <7.20 is ≈2%.
- If 1 or 2 components of the CTG are abnormal, the risk of a pH <7.20 is ≈20%.
- If 3–4 components of the CTG are abnormal, the risk of a pH <7.20 is ≈50%.

 If you're thinking you might be needing to do a FBS, its probably time to be doing it.

Place the mother in lithotomy with a 15° lateral tilt (or the left lateral position if approaching full dilatation). Insert an amnioscope appropriate for the dilatation and dry the scalp with a sponge or swab on long sponge-holders. Spray the scalp with ethyl chloride to induce hyperaemia and cover with a thin layer of paraffin jelly (so that the blood will form a blob and not run). Use the blade to make a small nick in the scalp and touch the blob with the capillary tube. Try not to touch the scalp directly (occludes the tube) and avoid admixture with any maternal blood in the vagina. Take three samples if possible to ensure consistency of results.

Fetal scalp pH correlates very poorly with Apgar scores. It is common practice to deliver if the pH is <7.20, although it may be the rate of fall in pH rather than the absolute value which is relevant.

- Only 15% of babies with pH < 7.1 have an Apgar score of <7 at 5 minutes.
- Only 20% of babies with an Apgar score of <7 at 5 minutes have a pH <7.1 (Lancet 1982;i:494).

Long-term prognosis following 'fetal distress'

Of those babies with an Apgar score <3 at 10 minutes, two-thirds die within 1 year. Of the survivors, 80% are normal. Neonatal encephalopathy is a better guide to long-term outlook than are Apgar scores:

- Grade 1. Hyperalert, decreased tone, jittery, dilated pupils: usually resolves in 24 hours.
- Grade 2. Lethargic, weak suck, fits: 15–27% chance of severe sequelae.
- Grade 3. Flaccid, no suck, no Moro reflex, prolonged fits: nearly 100% chance of severe sequelae.

The prognosis is generally good if the baby does not develop grade 3 encephalopathy, or if grade 2 encephalopathy lasts <5 days. Further clinical evaluation may be available from EEG (the incidence of death or handicap is low if the EEG is normal or near normal), CT (the prognosis is good if the CT is normal or shows only patchy hypodensities) or USS (the incidence of impairment correlates with intracerebral hypoechogenic areas of necrosis). The incidence of cerebral palsy in term infants has not changed with 'improved' obstetric care, and probably <10% of cases are due to intrapartum events (Br Med J 1999:1054).

HAEMORRHAGE (see also PV Spotting, p. 55)

> This may be rapidly fatal. Prepare by ensuring that there is a protocol/drill in the unit and that there is a process to get blood quickly. Beware of the tendency to underestimate the severity of the bleeding. Mobilize help from obstetricians, anaesthetists, midwives, the blood transfusion service, porters and senior haematologists. You cannot have enough help.

Antepartum haemorrhage

 Do not carry out an antenatal PV examination until placenta praevia has been excluded. No PV until no PP.

This is defined as PV bleeding at >24 weeks and occurs in 3% of all pregnancies.

- *Abruption*. There is an increased risk of recurrence in subsequent pregnancies.
- *Placenta praevia* (see p. 55). Placenta praevia caesarean sections should be supervised/performed by a senior obstetrician.
- *Uterine rupture* (see p. 82). This occurs only very rarely.
- *Vasa praevia* (beware when a succenturiate lobe is diagnosed). There is rapid fetal distress and usually no time for App's test. (Two drops of vaginal blood to 10 ml of 0.1 M KOH, and two drops of maternal blood to a further 10 ml of 0.1 M KOH. The maternal tube remains brown, the fetal tube turns pink.)

Management

- Carry out maternal and fetal assessment, including an accurate calculation of the gestation time, CTG and USS for the placental site.
- Consider delivery and the method of delivery (note there is an increased risk of PPH). Induction of labour is often relatively easy, although there is a small risk that the delay may exacerbate fetal distress and any coagulopathy.
- Gain IV access with *two* Grey Venflons. Take bloods for: Hb, H'CRIT, platelets, clotting and crossmatch RCC (the number of units depends on the volume lost).
- Give crystalloid or colloid (Haemaccel or Gelofusine, *not* Dextran) as required (note that there is controversy about this; Br Med J 1998;317:235).
- See Further Management of Haemorrhage, below.

Postpartum haemorrhage

This is defined as >500 ml blood. It is commoner in grand multiparity, multiple pregnancy, fibroids, praevia, following an APH and in those with a past history of PPH.

The PPH is *primary* if it occurs <24 hours postdelivery. It is *secondary* if it occurs 24 hours to 6 weeks postdelivery. Primary PPH is due to:

- in 90% of cases, atony ± retained products of conception;
- in 7% of cases, trauma;
- in 3% of cases, coagulation problem (usually DIC);
- multiple causes may be present.

[handwritten margin note: Tone / Trauma / Tissue / Thrombin]

Management

- Rub up a contraction by abdominal massage.
- Gain IV access with *two* Grey Venflons. Take bloods for Hb, H'CRIT, platelets, clotting and crossmatch RCC (the number of units depends on the volume lost).
- Give Syntocinon 10 IU stat. IV and then 20 IU in 500 ml Hartman's solution at 125 ml/h or faster if required.
- Give crystalloid or colloid (Haemaccel or Gelofusine, *not* Dextran) as required (note that there is controversy about this; Br Med J 1998;317:235).
- Remove the placenta. Try continuous cord traction initially. If the placenta is retained, a regional block or GA will be required, but pethidine 50 mg IV with midazolam 2–10 mg IV may be used if absolutely necessary. If there is placenta accreta and there is no bleeding *do not attempt any further removal*, but leave and manage conservatively. If bleeding, hysterectomy may be required.
- Give further oxytocics, e.g. Syntocinon 20 IU IV stat, ergometrine 0.5 mg IV or carboprost (Hemabate) 250 µg (= 1 ml = 1 ampoule) IM or intramyometrial (*not IV*) with further doses 90 minutes apart (or at least more than 15 minutes apart). Hemabate is contraindicated with cardiac, pulmonary, renal or

hepatic disease. Side-effects include GI upset, particularly diarrhoea, and pyrexia. Consider also a gemeprost pessary PV.

- Under GA, check for vaginal or cervical lacerations with general or spinal analgesia ('walk the cervix' with Rampley's sponge-holding forceps). In unexplained PPH, laparotomy should not be unduly delayed.
- See Further Management of Haemorrhage, below.

Further management of haemorrhage

- Consider a CVP if the clotting is normal.
- Transfuse, ideally with warmed blood under pressure (filtration not usually necessary). O-Negative or group-specific uncrossmatched blood may be used in an extreme emergency. Each unit of RCC ≈260 ml. Give 10 ml of 10% calcium chloride (or gluconate) IV over 10 minutes for every 6 U of RCC (sodium citrate preservative binds calcium). Major transfusion may lead to hyperkalaemia.
- Correct the coagulation defects of DIC with:
  — FFP (usually in packs of 300 ml), which contains clotting factors.
  — Cryoprecipitate. This is prepared from FFP and is a rich source of fibrinogen, factor VIII and von Willebrand factor. Use if the fibrinogen is low.
  — Platelet concentrate (needs to be ABO and Rhesus compatible). This is stored at room temperature (do not refrigerate) and is generally only required if the platelets are $<50 \times 10^9/l$ in the presence of active bleeding (note damaged transfused platelets may aggravate DIC).
  — There is no indication for tranxenamic acid (risk of fibrin deposition in kidneys) or aprotinin (may also have anticoagulation properties) in DIC.
- Hysterectomy (or subtotal hysterectomy) may be indicated, especially if there is a non-lower-segment uterine rupture or placenta accreta. Internal iliac artery ligation is only likely to be suitable for atony, is of less use with placenta accreta and is of no use for uterine lacerations. Uterine packing is an option for atony, but may in itself prevent an adequate uterine contraction and, therefore, haemostasis.
- Radiologically directed arterial embolization is also an option for uncontrolled haemorrhage.
- See also Acute Renal Failure (p. 98) and Adult Respiratory Distress Syndrome (p. 99) if appropriate.

UTERINE RUPTURE

This may occur with a previous caesarean section (the risk with a lower segment incision is <1%, and that with a classical or De Lee incision is 5–10%). It may also occur with obstructed labour in multiparous patients and with use of prostaglandins or Syntocinon. It is very rare in primigravidae.

Symptoms and signs

Rupture may occur prelabour or in labour. When it occurs during labour:

- Classically, there is maternal tachycardia, shock, cessation of contractions, disappearance of the presenting part from the pelvis and fetal distress. Pain may be minimal or may be severe and there is variable PV bleeding (bleeding is intraperitoneal if there is a complete rupture) or haematuria.
- Rupture may present postpartum with a continued trickle of bleeding in the absence of another cause.

Management of antenatal rupture

- Set up an IV infusion.
- Crossmatch 6 U of RCC (see Haemorrhage, p. 81).
- Perform an immediate laparotomy under GA or rapid spinal block for delivery. The majority of spontaneous ruptures (85%) require hysterectomy, but more than 65% of ruptured scars can be repaired. Uterine artery ligation may be of limited use in uterine rupture or scar dehiscence.
- Antibiotic cover with amoxicillin 500 mg IV (or cefuroxime 750 mg IV TID if penicillin allergic) and gentamicin (see p. 104) is advised.

CORD PROLAPSE

> This occurs especially when membranes rupture or are ruptured with a high presenting part. It is also more likely to occur with twins, polyhydramnios, breech or transverse lie. Prolapse following ARM is, by definition, iatrogenic. Abdominal palpation should precede artificial rupture of the membranes (ARM).

Management

- If the cord is palpated before ARM ('cord presentation'), proceed to caesarean section.
- If the cord is prolapsed:
  — Displace the presenting part upwards with a hand and keep it up. Do not handle the cord itself as there is a risk of spasm, leading to profound bradycardia ± asystole (beware erroneous diagnosis of IUD).
  — If the cervix is fully dilated and easy delivery is anticipated, carry out an immediate forceps or ventouse delivery (for a second twin, breech extraction may be considered, see p. 53).
  — If the cervix is not fully dilated, then instruct the patient to adopt the heel–elbow position (kneeling with head down) and transfer her to theatre for an immediate caesarean section under GA or rapid spinal anaesthesia.

MALPRESENTATIONS AND MALPOSITIONS

Occipitoposterior (occipitofrontal diameter 11 cm) (Fig. 3.6) 90%.
Although the head usually rotates to occipitoanterior in normal labour,
some arrest in the transverse position and a small proportion (≈10%) rotate
to occipitoposterior (OP) (Fig. 3.6). There are usually longer first and second
stages of labour, with an increased chance of requiring a caesarean section,
rotational forceps or ventouse delivery. If still OP and undelivered despite
second stage pushing, a low/midcavity OP delivery, manual rotation,
rotational ventouse, or Keilland's rotational forceps delivery will be
required.

Breech (see also p. 40)

> ⚠ **Do not confuse a face presentation with a breech
> presentation on vaginal examination.**

The first stage is managed with caution. The role of epidural is controversial
– its use may facilitate manipulation of the fetus, but its presence may inhibit

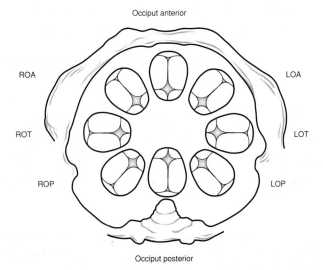

Fig. 3.6 Position of scalp sutures on vaginal examination.

the desire to push, which is so important in breech delivery. Augmentation must only be used if disproportion has been excluded, and even then with caution. There is no contraindication to a fetal 'scalp' clip being applied to the breech, providing care is taken to avoid genital injury.

The bitrochanteric diameter engages the pelvic brim in the transverse (much as the sagittal suture is transverse with cephalic presentation). As the breech descends, it rotates to AP and advances over the perineum with pushing (Fig. 3.7). Perform an episiotomy. Resist the temptation to pull. If the breech is frank, flex the knees to deliver the legs, and wait for the body to advance further. The anterior shoulder is delivered under the symphysis. If this is not possible, the posterior shoulder may be delivered first by rotating the back 180° (anteriorly), bringing the shoulder anteriorly under the symphysis. The baby is then rotated 180° back again (again with the back anteriorly) for the remaining shoulder (Lovset's manoeuvre). Let the breech hang to flex the head, then lift the whole body up vertically by the legs (an assistant should hold the legs). The head can then be delivered by outlet forceps. Alternatively, by gently putting the index finger of one hand in the baby's mouth (avoid traction on the jaw) and the index and middle fingers of the other hand on the occiput, the head can be delivered by flexion (Mauriceau Smellie Veit).

Should the head of a preterm breech become entrapped behind an incompletely dilated cervix, it should first be flexed as far as possible to narrow the presenting diameter. Failing this, the options are then to:

- Incise the cervix at the 4 and 8 o'clock positions (risking massive, potentially fatal maternal haemorrhage).
- Push the fetus back up (very difficult) and perform a caesarean section.
- Use nitroglycerine. A number of case reports have shown that following 100 µg IV bolus intravenous nitroglycerin there is a sudden transient cervicouterine relaxation within 45–90 seconds, lasting about 1 minute (repeat 100 µg IV bolus 2–3 minutes later if required). Nitroglycerine is contraindicated with uncorrected hypovolaemia, severe anaemia (Hb < 6 g/dl), increased intracranial pressure, constrictive pericarditis/pericardial tamponade and hypersensitivity to GTN. Haemodynamic monitoring, a rapidly running IV infusion and immediately available ephedrine (see p. 73) are mandatory prior to the use of nitroglycerine. (Nitroglycerine may also be considered when uterine relaxation is required during a difficult caesarean section.)

Face presentation (submentobregmatic diameter 9.5 cm)

Most engage in the transverse position, and 90% rotate to mentoanterior so that the head is born with flexion. If mentoposterior, a caesarean section will be required unless the baby is very pre-term or there is IUD.

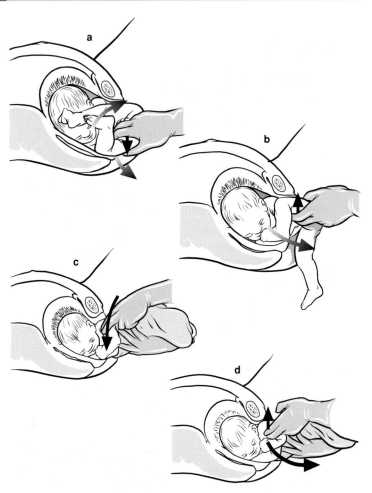

Fig. 3.7 a Flexion of left knee with a frank breech presenting left sacrotransverse. **b** Flexion of right knee. **c** Flexion of the left arm for **d** delivery under the symphysis pubis.

Brow presentation (mentovertical diameter 13 cm)

The supraorbital ridges and the bridge of the nose are palpable. The head may flex to become a vertex presentation or extend to face presentation in early labour. If the brow presentation persists or there is no cervical dilatation, a caesarean section will be required. Examine 2 hourly. Do not use Syntocinon.

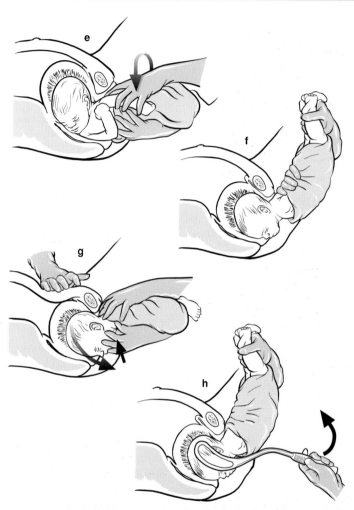

e Rotation of the back anteriorly allows delivery of the posterior shoulder. **f** Lifting the body after allowing the breech to hang. **g** Mauriceau Smellie Veit for head delivery. **h** Alternative delivery of the head with forceps.

Transverse/oblique lie

This usually occurs in multiparous women and is associated with multiple pregnancy, preterm labour and polyhydramnios. It may also occur with an abnormal uterus or placenta praevia. Vaginal delivery is not possible and there is a risk of cord prolapse. Consider prelabour ECV ±induction, or elective caesarean section. Transverse lie (±arm presentation) following SRM is an indication for urgent caesarean section, which may require a vertical uterine incision (i.e. classical or De Lees).

OPERATIVE DELIVERY

> There is no substitute for direct hands-on experience, and new techniques should only be tried under close experienced supervision.

Forceps delivery

There are three main types of forceps:

- Low-cavity outlet forceps (e.g. Wrigley's), which are short and light.
- Midcavity forceps (e.g. Haig Ferguson, Neville Barnes, Simpson's) for when sagittal suture is AP (usually OA).
- Keilland's forceps for rotational delivery (the reduced pelvic curve allows rotation about the axis of the handle). Senior experience is required and details are not given here.

The most common indications are presumed fetal distress or second-stage delay. The cervix must be fully dilated, the head at spines or below and analgesia satisfactory (perineal infiltration and pudendal blocks usually suffice for midcavity and ventouse deliveries, but regional analgesia is required for Keilland's). Often the most difficult part is identifying the fetal position accurately (regional analgesia may occasionally be required). If there is a suspicion from palpation of the sutures that the baby is transverse, it is often helpful to try and feel for an ear anteriorly under the symphysis pubis (this is painful).

Low or midcavity non-rotational forceps (Fig. 3.8)

- Check abdominal palpation. The mother should be placed in the lithotomy position with her bottom just over the edge of the bed (the bottom half of the bed often lifts away). Clean and drape. Empty the bladder. Recheck that the cervix is fully dilated, and that you are sure about the position and station of the head.
- Insert a pudendal block. (Draw up 20 ml of 1% lignocaine. Pass the pudendal needle through the sacrospinous ligament and, after withdrawing to ensure that the injection is not intravascular, inject 7 ml of 1% lignocaine behind each ligament.) Use the remaining 6 ml of lignocaine to the infiltrate the perineum (in the 7 o'clock position).
- Discretely assemble the forceps in front of the perineum before application, ensuring that the pelvic curve will be sitting over the malar aspect of the

baby's head, convex towards the baby's face. The handle which lies in the left hand is inserted to the mother's left side by placing the right hand into the vagina and slipping the blade between your hand and baby's head between contractions. Use opposite hands for the right blade and ensure that the forceps lock easily. Once locked, the operator should not be able to insert a finger within the 'window' of the cephalic curve.

● Apply traction, pulling initially downwards at an angle of ≈60° (maternal pelvis to your pelvis if sitting), with the direction of traction becoming horizontal and then upwards as the baby's head advances over the perineum. It is usual to perform an episiotomy as the vulva stretches, but occasionally this may not be necessary with a low cavity lift out in a parous woman. Remove the forceps after delivery of the baby's head, check for cord, wait for restitution of the head, and deliver the anterior shoulder with downward traction (it is not necessary to wait for a further contraction to deliver the shoulder). Give Syntocinon 10 IU IM. Deliver the placenta with continuous cord traction *after* the uterus contracts, and repair the episiotomy and any tears.

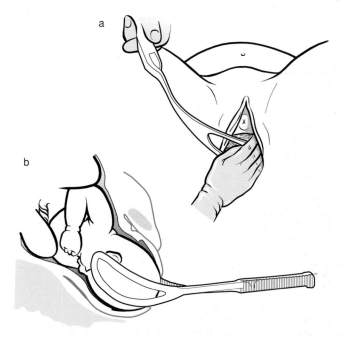

Fig. 3.8 a Application of forceps. **b** Correction application prior to traction.

Manual rotation

This is a very useful adjunct to malposition. It may be possible to rotate the fetal head to OA using digital pressure on the sutures (usually the lambdoid sutures). Some operators prefer to rotate during a contraction in order to minimize the risk of pushing the head up out of the pelvis.

Ventouse delivery (Fig. 3.9)

Ventouse delivery may be associated with less maternal trauma, but this is controversial (Br J Obstet Gynaecol 1996:608). The same criteria apply to ventouse delivery as to forceps. It is traditional to use a silastic cup for outlet deliveries, a metal cup for midcavity deliveries and an OP cup for transverse and posterior malpositions. The cup is ideally placed in the midline overlying, or just anterior to, the posterior fontanelle (see Fig. 3.9a). Apply suction initially at $0.2 \, kg/cm^2$, check that vaginal skin has not been included and then immediately increase the suction to $0.8 \, kg \, cm^2$. Apply traction downwards, as for a forceps delivery. Delivery is much more likely to be successful if traction is timed with contractions and maternal effort. If standing, it is useful to place one foot close to the patient and one foot behind you to avoid, in case of cup detachment, an embarrassing collapse on the floor. The risk of significant fetal injury is increased with the use of metal cups (rather than silastic), and the duration of application.

Caesarean section

Maternal mortality is higher for emergency than for elective section. Overall there is also significant morbidity from thromboembolic disease, haemorrhage and infection. Lower uterine segment caesarean section is by far the most commonly used and has a lower rate of subsequent uterine rupture, together with better healing and fewer postoperative complications. A classical caesarean section will provide better access for a transverse lie following ruptured membranes, or with very vascular anterior placenta praevias, very preterm fetuses, or large lower segment fibroids.

Be fully aware of the labour ward's emergency procedure for contacting the anaesthetist, theatre staff, midwives and paediatricians. All these people will need to know the degree of urgency and the specific indication for delivery, in particular the anaesthetist to decide between regional and general anaesthesia.

Insert a venflon, send a group and save (or crossmatch if there is an increased risk of bleeding) and give 30 ml of 0.3 M sodium citrate (to reduce the incidence of Mendelson's syndrome, see p. 104). Elective sections should also be given ranitidine 150 mg PO 12 and 2 hours before the operation. *Ensure that you have thought about appropriate thromboprophylaxis (see p. 149) and antibiotic prophylaxis.*

● The table should be tilted 15° to the left side. Check that the lie is longitudinal. Catheterize after anaesthesia.

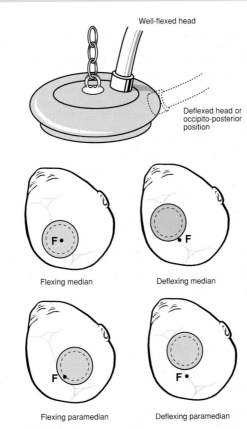

Well-flexed head

Deflexed head or
occipito-posterior
position

a

Flexing median

Deflexing median

Flexing paramedian

Deflexing paramedian

b

Fig. 3.9 a Vacuum extractor cups for a well-flexed head, and for application to a deflexed head
or occipitoposterior position. **b** Correct and incorrect ventouse cup application. F, The ideal
point for traction. Failure to deliver is higher with the other positions, particularly deflexing
paramedian.

● Use the scalpel to perform a lower abdominal transverse incision, cutting
through the fat to the rectus sheath overlying the rectus abdominus
muscles. Cut through the sheath for 1 cm or so either side of midline,
still using the scalpel, and then use the scissors to extend this laterally.
Dissect under the sheath above and below using a combination of sharp
and blunt dissection and then explore through the rectus muscles in the
midline to find the peritoneum. Open the peritoneum with care (high up)
*making certain that you are not cutting into bladder or bowel, particularly at an
advanced cervical dilatation.*

- Once through, open fully with scissors, insert a retractor into the lower part of the wound, lift up the visceral peritoneum over the lower segment with toothed dissectors and divide with scissors. Use the scissors to divide this laterally and push the bladder down before making a transverse lower segment incision. The anterior lower segment is the portion of the uterus below the reflection of the peritoneum (i.e. below the line along which the peritoneum is firmly adherent). If the bladder is densely adherent to the uterus (e.g. after previous caesareans) it may be better to make a transverse incision above the bladder rather than risk unnecessary bladder trauma.

- Encourage the baby's head through the incision with firm, fundal pressure from the assistant (it may occasionally be helpful to use Wrigley's forceps). If the baby is breech, apply traction to the pelvis by placing a finger behind each flexed hip, or find an extended leg to pull and deliver with fundal pressure from the assistant. Encourage the assistant to 'follow' the head down, as this promotes flexion. If transverse, also try to find a leg (*do not pull an arm*).

After delivery, give Syntocinon 10 IU IV stat. and *wait for the uterus to contract* before delivering the placenta. Attain haemostasis with straight artery forceps. Check the uterus is empty and close with two layers of dissolving suture (e.g. Vicryl) to the uterus, one layer to the sheath and one layer to the skin. There is no need to close the peritoneum.

SHOULDER DYSTOCIA

> Prompt, calm action is vital. Make the diagnosis after failure to deliver shoulders with the *first* downward pull of the head. The shoulders are stuck in the AP plane with the anterior shoulder behind the symphysis pubis (Br J Obstet Gynaecol 1998:815)

Management
Use PALE SISTER (see Box opposite)

Postdelivery
Beware PPH. Check the baby for asphyxia, brachial plexus injury, fractured clavicle and fractured ribs. Regarding the next delivery, one series reviewed 51 deliveries (Br J Obstet Gynaecol 1994:713): five had an elective caesarean section; of the 42 that had vaginal deliveries, five had further shoulder dystocia (i.e. ≈10%, compared to the incidence in the normal population of 0.15–1.3%), although there were no episodes of fetal trauma or death.

P **Prepare**. Have a plan, practise it and ensure that the team knows the plan.

A **Assistance**. Send for experienced help, but start management immediately.

L **Legs into McRoberts**. Femora abducted, rotated outwards and flexed (such that the thighs touch the abdomen). This straightens the sacrum relative to the lumbar spine, rotating the symphysis anteriorly and allows the anterior shoulder to enter the pelvis.

E **Episiotomy**. Make it large.

S **Suprapubic pressure**. An assistant should apply suprapubic pressure with 'CPR' hand posture over the anterior shoulder, both laterally towards the direction the baby is facing and posteriorly to rotate it under the symphysis, while gentle traction is applied from below ± rocking technique. Abandon after 30–60 seconds.

I **Internal rotation**. Continue traction and insert a hand to push the anterior shoulder forwards with counter pressure on the posterior clavicle to rotate the trunk to oblique. Abandon after 30–60 seconds.

S **Screw manoeuvre**. Apply pressure to the posterior aspect of the posterior shoulder, attempting to place the shoulder into oblique. This may disimpact the anterior shoulder. If this fails, continue through 180° – the anterior shoulder is now posterior. Abandon after 30–60 seconds.

T **Try recovering posterior arm**. Attempt to deliver the posterior shoulder by pulling the posterior arm down, flexing it across the chest. Abandon after 30–60 seconds.

E **Extreme measures**. The choices are:

- Try the above again.
- Fracture the clavicle (it may already be fractured after the above manoeuvres).
- Push the baby's head back up and perform a caesarean section (Zavanelli Manoeuvre).
- Perform a symphysiotomy:
  - Inject 10 ml of 1% lignocaine plain to the skin over the symphysis pubis.
  - Do not abduct the legs >80° (use two assistants to hold the legs).
  - Insert a foley catheter into the urethra, sliding it to one side out of the way with one hand.
  - Using the other hand, insert a scalpel under the skin, blade away from you, and make one stab incision approximately at the junction between the lower third and the upper two thirds of the symphysis. When the scalpel tip is just felt by the hand supporting the urethra, rotate the scalpel up towards the mother's head, thus dividing the upper two-thirds of the symphysis. Take the scalpel out, rotate 180°, reinsert and partially divide the lower third of the symphysis in a similar way.

R **Repair, record details, relax**. Explain to patient. Make comprehensive notes.

RETAINED PLACENTA

> With oxytocics and continuous cord traction, 97% of third stages are complete by 10 minutes. The physiological third stage should be less than 30 minutes, but waiting until 60 minutes (rather than 30) halves the number of women requiring anaesthesia. Retained placenta is more likely if a previous manual removal has been required. There is an increased risk of PPH.

Management

- Use continuous cord traction while protecting the fundus with the other hand to prevent uterine inversion.
- If not delivered:
  — Carry out a VE to ensure that the placenta is not sitting in the vagina. If nearly out, it may be possible to remove it with entonox or midazolam 2–10 mg IV stat. (caution: respiratory depression, see p. 104).
  — If not, set up an IVI and crossmatch 2 u of RCC. Give prophylactic antibiotics (e.g. augmentin 1.2 g IV stat.).
  — Use a spinal or epidural block or GA for manual removal in theatre. If the placenta does not separate, it may be a placenta accreta. If not bleeding, *do not attempt any further removal*, but leave and manage conservatively. If the patient is bleeding a hysterectomy may be required (see Haemorrhage, p. 80).
  — When the cavity is empty, give oxytocin 10 iu IV stat.

UTERINE INVERSION

> This is usually an iatrogenic problem. Suspect uterine inversion if there is profound shock without an obvious cause. The inversion may be partial or total.

Management

- Do not detach the placenta until the uterus is replaced and contracted.
- If the prolapse is easily reducible, try to reduce it.
- Start antishock measures with IV access and colloid.
- If reduction is unsuccessful, use hydrostatic reduction (O'Sullivan's): *exclude perforation* by clinical inspection. The inverted uterus is held within the vagina by the operator and the introitus sealed with the two hands of an assistant. Infuse 2 litres of warm saline rapidly (e.g. with 1000 ml bags of saline through a silastic ventouse cup, urological Y giving set, or with a funnel and anaesthetic machine scavenging tubing).
- Once corrected, give syntometrine 1 ml IM stat.
- If all this fails, consider laparotomy. Hysterectomy may be necessary.

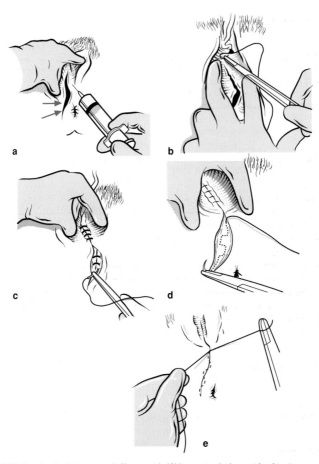

Fig. 3.10 Repair of episiotomy. **a** Infiltrate with 1% lignocaine (unless epidural in situ or perineum infiltrated prior to delivery). Maximum lignocaine is 4 mg/kg (*NB: not 4 ml/kg*) without adrenaline and 8 mg/kg with adrenaline (e.g. 28 ml of 1% plain lignocaine in a 70 kg woman). Polyglycolic acid is the preferred suture material (Br J Obstet Gynaecol 1998:441), e.g. No. 1 gauge for the vagina and perineal body, and 2/0 for the skin. **b** Find the apex of the vaginal incision or tear and place the first suture above this level (*caution:* rectum posterior to vaginal wall). **c** Use a continuous locking suture to oppose the vaginal wall, continuing until the hymenal edges are opposed. The suture can then be tied or, more simply, locked, and the needle threaded between the opposed vaginal edges a few centimetres back ready to close the perineal body. **d** The perineal body sutures should be interrupted, and then a continuous finer suture used for the skin. It is possible that not closing the skin (i.e. leaving the skin edges approximately 5 mm apart) reduces postnatal pain (Br J Obstet Gynaecol 1998:435). **e** Check instruments and swabs (a common cause of litigation in obstetrical and gynaecological practice). Carry out a PR to make sure that sutures have not penetrated the rectum.

EPISIOTOMY REPAIR

See Figure 3.10.

POSTNATAL PROBLEMS

> There is evidence that puerperal morbidity is generally high. This area of care is often neglected, and problems may become chronic. At 3 months at least 20% of women are suffering stress incontinence, up to 20% report constipation and 4% are unable to control flatus or faeces.

Puerperal pyrexia

This is defined as a temperature >38°C on any occasion in the first 14 days after delivery or miscarriage (a slight fever is not uncommon in the first 24 hours). Pyrexia is usually due to urinary or genital infections (including endometritis), but may also be related to infection in the chest or breast. DVT and PTE must not be forgotten. After a full clinical examination (including breasts, legs, perineum and abdominal palpation of the uterus) send an MSU and endocervical ± wound swab for culture. If there is any suggestion of a chest infection, also send sputum for culture. Send blood cultures if the patient is systemically unwell.

> **Remember**
>
> Carry out appropriate investigations if there is any suspicion of a venous thromboembolic disease (see p. 146).

In general, if the patient is well and the temperature only mildly elevated, conservative treatment may be warranted. If the source of infection is not clear, treat with either co-amoxiclav (e.g. Augmentin) 2 tablets PO TID (or 1.2 g IV TID) or with a combination of amoxicillin 500 mg QID PO (or IV) and metronidazole 400 mg PO TID (500 mg IV). Treat breast infections with flucloxacillin 500 mg PO QID. Breast-feeding should continue.

Anaemia

The incidence of postnatal anaemia is 25–30%. It is reasonable simply to treat nonsymptomatic anaemia with oral iron, reserving transfusion for those with troublesome symptomatology.

Breast problems

Two-thirds of women will have some problem, including nipple pain, engorgement, cracks and bleeding. These can largely be prevented by proper advice regarding positioning of the baby's mouth and supportive counselling. Mastitis is frequently due to a blocked duct, but can occur secondary to infection (e.g. *Staphylococcus aureus*, see above). Breast feeding should continue.

Superficial thrombophlebitis
This affects about 1% of women. There is a painful, erythematous and tender (usually varicose) vein. Treat with support stockings and give anti-inflammatory drugs (e.g. ibuprofen 400 mg TID PO).

Secondary haemorrhage
This is defined as bleeding between 24 hours and 6 weeks postnatally. It is usually due to infection or retained products of conception, rarely to a vulval haematoma, very rarely to caesarean scar dehiscence and only exceptionally to trophoblastic disease. Check P, BP, temperature, uterine tenderness, haemoglobin and an endocervical swab. In practice, the decision is usually between giving antibiotics or arranging for an evacuation of retained products with antibiotic cover under anaesthesia (this can often be done digitally, particularly in the first week, without the need to instrument the uterus and risk perforation). Clinical judgement is important, perhaps giving antibiotics in the first instance if the bleeding is not severe, and arranging an evacuation if it does not settle. Do not rush into arranging an initial USS as many normal women have asymptomatic retained products after entirely normal deliveries and one is then tempted to carry out an unnecessary and potentially hazardous uterine evacuation.

Episiotomy breakdown
This is common, but long-term problems are rare. If the wound is clean, consider re-suturing. If there is any suggestion of infection, however, it is probably better to allow healing by secondary intention. Keep the perineum clean (e.g. baths or bidet BD) and consider antibiotics for infection.

The postnatal examination
This takes place at 6 weeks and should be a chance to review the delivery, answer any doubts or questions and place these in context for future deliveries. Also:

- How is the baby?
- How is the mother coping (tiredness, depression)?
- Check maternal Hb.
- Check cervical smear, if appropriate.
- Arrange contraception (see p. 162).
- Has intercourse been resumed? Any problems? (See p. 211).

ACUTE MEDICAL PROBLEMS

ACUTE RENAL FAILURE

> Acute renal failure is characterized initially by <u>oliguria</u> (usually <400 ml in 24 hours) ± a <u>rising creatinine</u> and <u>potassium</u>, and <u>may last days or weeks</u>. There follows a <u>polyuric phase</u>, which may also <u>last days</u> or <u>weeks</u> (passing up to 10 l/day), and then finally, but not always, recovery.

Causes

- *Pre-renal*: e.g. haemorrhage (see p. 80), sepsis (Gram-negative septicaemia, see p. 104).
- *Renal*: e.g. pre-eclampsia/HELLP syndrome (see p. 133), eclampsia or drugs. Renal injury (i.e. the potentially reversible acute tubular necrosis, or cortical necrosis which is irreversible) may occur secondary to pre-renal problems
- *Postrenal*: e.g. bilateral ureteric obstruction following surgery.

Investigations

Check U&E, serum osmolality, $Ca^{2+}PO^{4-}$, albumin, creatinine, LFTs, coagulation screen, FBC, ESR, blood cultures and ABGs. Send urine for microscopy and osmolality. Arrange a CXR (? fluid overload), a renal USS (? obstruction, renal abnormality) and an ECG.

Management

- Involve physicians at an early stage.
- Identify and correct the underlying cause.
- Identify and correct pre-renal failure (hypovolaemia) with the aid of CVP monitoring.
- If $\uparrow K^+$, there may be tented T waves with a prolonged QRS. There is a risk of arrhythmias:
  — if >6.8 mmol/l, give 50 ml 50% dextrose IV and 10 units actrapid IV over 30 min;
  — if >8.0 mmol/l, also give 10 ml 10% calcium gluconate, slow IV (cardioprotective effect).
- If $\downarrow Na^+$, the patient may become drowsy, unconscious or may fit:
  — if 125–132 mmol/l, fluid restrict;
  — if <125 mmol/l, probably need dialysis.
- Treat acidosis if HCO^{3-} on ABG sample <12 mmol/l. Use 8.4% sodium bicarbonate (1 ml = 1 mmol) and aim for an HCO^{3-} level of 18–22 mmol/l:
  — Dose in ml (slow IV) = $(15 - pHCO^{3-}) \times$ weight (kg) $\times 0.6$
- Treat $\downarrow Ca^{2+}$ only if symptomatic (carpopedal spasm, Chvostek's sign).

- Fluid input should = output of previous day + 500 ml + 200 ml per degree of raised temperature (°C).

  Give a low protein, high fat and high carbohydrate diet with low K^+ and Na^+. Consider dialysis if there is rapid deterioration, volume overload (±pulmonary oedema), uraemic symptoms (confusion, nausea, vomiting or pruritus), hyperkalaemia or acidosis despite the above measures.
- Critically review all pharmacological agents and reduce doses accordingly (e.g. $MgSO_4$, aminoglycosides).

ACUTE PULMONARY OEDEMA

> In obstetrics, the commonest cause is fluid overload, particularly in the presence of pre-eclampsia (see also ARDS, below).

Management

- Identify and correct the underlying cause.
- Sit the patient upright and attach an O_2 saturation monitor, if available.
- Check ABGs and CXR.
- Give high-flow O_2 therapy.
- Give frusemide 50 mg bolus IV.
- Give morphine 5–10 mg bolus IV.
- A CVP line may assist with ongoing management, particularly in pre-eclampsia.
- Review drug therapy. Stop or avoid β-blockers (replace with hydralazine).

ADULT RESPIRATORY DISTRESS SYNDROME (ARDS)

> A cascade of increased pulmonary vascular permeability, loss of lung volume, reduced compliance, shunting and arterial hypoxaemia which may be secondary to aspiration, DIC, pre-eclampsia, haemorrhage, hydatidiform mole, sepsis, overtransfusion or amniotic fluid embolism. More than 70% of cases are due to a combination of causes.

- *Stage 1.* There is hyperventilation with adequate arterial oxygenation.
- *Stage 2.* In the latent period, the respiratory rate is >20/min and there are minor auscultatory changes of alveolar and interstitial oedema. There are also minor radiographic changes and hypoxaemia with a respiratory alkalosis. Treat with an O_2 mask and monitor with a pulse oximeter (aiming for >90% saturation).

- *Stage 3.* There is respiratory failure refractory to high-flow O_2, usually occurring 24–72 hours after the initial onset of symptoms, with dyspnoea, tachypnoea, $\downarrow O_2$ and organization of hyaline membrane. There is bilateral diffuse infiltration on the CXR. Ventilate using positive peak end expiratory pressure ±Swan–Ganz catheter monitoring. There is no indication for prophylactic antibiotics per se, or mannitol.
- *Stage 4.* Irreversible shunting, severe refractory hypoxaemia and hypercapnia with metabolic and respiratory acidosis eventually lead to cardiac arrest.

Pitfalls of treatment

- Avoid fluid overload, especially with colloid.
- Invasive ITU monitoring with help from the anaesthetists is mandatory.
- High oxygen concentrations may contribute to further lung injury; therefore use the minimum O_2 concentration necessary to achieve >90% saturation.

AMNIOTIC FLUID EMBOLISM

This has a high maternal mortality (up to 80%) and is associated with multiparity, precipitate labour, uterine stimulation and caesarean section. Clinically there is sudden dyspnoea, fetal distress and hypotension followed within minutes by cardiorespiratory arrest ± seizures. It is often followed by haemorrhage from DIC and uterine atony, and may lead to ARF and ARDS. Differentiation from pulmonary embolism, anaphylaxis, aspiration, MI and abruption may initially be difficult. It is often diagnosed by exclusion.

Management

- Carry out CPR with high-flow O_2 ± IPPV and consider urgent delivery.
- Insert two large-bore IV lines and infuse with crystalloid or colloid (note that there is controversy about this; Br Med J 1998;317:235), e.g. 2–4 units Haemaccel or Gelofusine until the BP is normal. Then stop the infusion to minimize the risk of ARDS.
- Check ABGs, U&E, LFT, FBC, clotting and crossmatch for 6 units of RCC.
- Correct any coagulopathy (see p. 82).
- As uterine atony is common, give oxytocics if delivered (see p. 81).
- Subsequent hypotension is usually due to cardiogenic shock; therefore consider transfer to the ITU for Swan–Ganz catheter monitoring and a dopamine infusion.
- If a central line is used, send a sample of blood from the right side of the heart to the pathology department to look for 'squamous cells' to support the diagnosis (absence of squames does not exclude the diagnosis). Sputum should also be sent to look for squamous cells.
- See ARDS (p. 99) or ARF (p. 98), if appropriate.

ANAPHYLAXIS

> An acute release of vasoactive substances leads to cyanosis, hypotension, wheezing, pallor, prostration and tachycardia.

Management

- Isolate the cause and remove (consider Latex allergy).
- Give high-flow O_2. If necessary, consider CPR or intubate for IPPV.
- Give adrenaline:
  - if severe, 5 ml 1:10 000 IM, or slow IV, or via an ET tube;
  - if mild/moderate, 0.5 ml 1:1000 SC or IM, repeating in 10 minutes if required.
- Insert a large-bore (14g) IV cannula and infuse 500–1000 ml colloid rapidly to re-expand the intravascular compartment.
- If wheeze is predominant, set up a salbutamol nebulizer 2.5 mg in 2.5 ml saline.
- Give hydrocortisone 100–200 mg IV over 2 minutes QID.
- Give chlorpheniramine 10 mg (i.e. 1 ml) IV over 1 minute.
- If there is deterioration, contact an anaesthetist.

CARDIORESPIRATORY ARREST

- If undelivered, consider lateral tilt.
- Commence basic and advanced cardiac life support (Fig. 3.11).
- Consider intrapartum causes (Table 3.2).

See also Table 3.3.

TABLE 3.2   Causes of sudden collapse

Cause	Features	Page
Amniotic fluid embolism	Is associated with multiparity, precipitate labour, uterine stimulation and caesarean section. There is *sudden dyspnoea, fetal distress* and *hypotension* followed within minutes by cardiorespiratory arrest ± seizures	100
Anaphylaxis	There may be *cyanosis, hypotension, wheezing, pallor*, prostration and tachycardia ± urticaria	101
Cerebrovascular accident	May be a past history of intracranial problems (e.g. previous subarachnoid haemorrhage). *Nausea and vomiting with headache.*	123
Eclampsia	There is a *tonic–clonic seizure* (differentiate from epilepsy and amniotic fluid embolism from history)	130
Myocardial infarct	May be a past history of heart disease. *Chest pain*	109
Tension pneumothorax	There is sudden onset of *pleuritic chest pain* (differentiate from pulmonary embolus) and diminished breath sounds	
Pulmonary embolism	There may be apprehension, *pleuritic chest pain, sudden dyspnoea,* cough, haemoptysis and collapse (differentiate from pneumothorax) ± antecedent risk factors	146
Uterine inversion	Occurs in the third stage only. It may lead to *profound hypotension.* (There may be only a partial inversion and, therefore, the diagnosis may not be obvious)	94

TABLE 3.3   Other emergencies

Emergency	Possible features	Page
Asthma	*Wheezing,* use of accessory muscles, previous history	143
Haemorrhage	May be antepartum or postpartum. Bleeding may be underestimated, particularly in *concealed abruption* (hard painful uterus) or *uterine rupture* (shock, cessation of contractions, disappearance of presenting part from pelvis and fetal distress)	80

ADULT ADVANCED LIFE SUPPORT

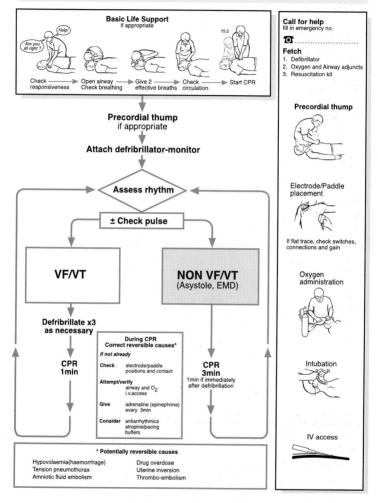

Fig. 3.11 Basic and advanced cardiac life support. (Based on the guidelines of the European Resuscitation Council, with permission.)

MENDELSON'S SYNDROME

This is due to inhalation of acid gastric contents. There is rapid onset of cyanosis, bronchospasm, tachycardia and pulmonary oedema. Differentiation from pulmonary embolus, congestive cardiac failure or amniotic fluid embolism may initially be difficult.

Prevention

- H_2 antagonist:
  — either ranitidine 150 mg PO 6 hours prior to operation;
  — or ranitidine 50 mg made up to 20 ml with normal saline IV given over 2 minutes closer to the operation.
- Sodium citrate 30 ml PO stat. prior to operation.
- Cricoid pressure with induction of GA.
- Aspiration of gastric contents before waking from emergency GA.

Management

- Put the patient's head down and turn it to one side.
- Aspirate the pharynx and give 100% O_2.
- Give aminophylline 5 mg/kg slowly IV (over 10 minutes).
- Give hydrocortisone 500 mg IV stat.
- Start ampicillin 500 mg QID IV and an aminoglycoside (e.g. gentamicin — give 4 mg/kg IV then daily at the same dose providing the gentamicin level 3 hours before the due dose is < 1 mg/l. If creatinine > 200 μmol/l, then dosage will need to be reduced).
- CXR, oximetry (or blood gases).
- Arrange physiotherapy
- Later, bronchoscopy under GA and aspiration of mucus plugs may be of benefit.

RESPIRATORY ARREST WITH OPIATES/ BENZODIAZEPINES/MgSO$_4$

Management

- Stop infusion of drug.
- Bag and mask with high-flow O_2, or intubate for IPPV.
- If *opiates*, give naloxone. This comes as 400 μg in 1 ml. Give 0.5 ml (200 μg) IV stat. then a further 0.25–0.5 ml (100–200 μg) as required.
- If *benzodiazepines*, give flumazenil. It comes as 5 ml of 100 μg/ml. Give 2 ml (200 μg) IV over 15 seconds, then 1 ml (100 μg) IV every 60 seconds to a maximum of 1 mg.
- If *MgSO$_4$*, see page 131.

SEPTICAEMIA

> Septicaemia may rapidly kill. It is often caused by endotoxins from Gram-negative bacilli, but is also caused by anaerobes and exotoxins from aerobic and anaerobic streptococci. There may be dehydration, hypotension, cyanosis, pallor, cold extremities, hypothermia and jaundice. ARDS may develop (see p. 99).

Investigations
FBC (WCC >15, platelets <50 ×10^9/l), clotting screen (DIC), U&E, LFTs ($\uparrow$bilirubin) and ABGs ($\downarrow p_aO_2$). There may also be haemoglobinuria (following haemolysis).

Management

- Give high-flow O_2.
- Give IV colloid and consider a CVP line.
- Start antibiotics (blind):
  - gentamicin (see dose p. 104) (as bacteriocidal, endotoxins may lead to initial deterioration),
  - and metronidazole 500 mg TID IV,
  - and ampicillin 500 mg QID IV.
- If there is a septic abortion, it is probably better to perform an ERPOC. If there is chorioamnionitis, deliver (vaginally or by caesarean section). A hysterectomy may have to be considered.
- Start heparin 5000 u BD or TID.
- See ARF (p. 98) and ARDS (p. 99), if appropriate.

TRANSFUSION REACTIONS

> **It is essential to check that the name and number of blood products corresponds to that of the patient prior to transfusion.**

Send all giving sets and bags to the BTS with 20 ml clotted blood.

TABLE 3.4   Transfusion reactions

Findings	Pathology	Management
Acute onset, becoming very unwell with fever and chills, shock, DIC, haemoglobinuria, oliguria, chest or back pains	ABO incompatibility → acute intravascular haemolysis (*rare*)	• Stop the transfusion and give oxygen • Support BP with normal saline or colloid • Take bloods: FBC, an EDTA for haptoglobulins (↑ in haemolysis), clotting (DIC), U&E (K⁺ rises in haemolysis) and LFTs (including bilirubin). Also send 20 ml of clotted blood and an EDTA tube to the BTS to confirm the diagnosis • ECG – risk of hyperkalaemia (see p. 119) • Catheterize for hourly urine volumes. Urine dipstick is usually positive for blood (haemoglobinuria). There is a risk of ARF (see p. 98). Give Frusemide 50 mg. If no diuresis, give 100 ml of 20% mannitol. If still no diuresis, consider CVP monitoring and involve renal physicians. Also consider dopamine IV infusion 2–5 mg/kg/h. • Repeat coagulation screens 2–4 hourly. Support with blood products if required (see p. 82) • If blood is still required, re-crossmatch. There is no increased risk of a second haemolytic reaction • See ARDS (p. 99) if appropriate
Uncomfortable, but not unwell. May have fever and chills	Antibodies to leucocytes or platelets (*common*)	• Slow or stop the transfusion • Give antipyretics, e.g. paracetamol 1 g PO QID • Consider leucocyte poor red cells if recurrent
Acute onset of urticaria or rarely of anaphylaxis	Antibodies to plasma → allergic reaction (*rare*)	• Stop the transfusion • See Anaphylaxis, p. 101 • Give washed red blood cells if recurrent
Late onset (days) of fever, anaemia, hyperbilirubinaemia, but remaining relatively well	Non-ABO, anti-RBC antibodies, e.g. Rhesus, Kell, Kidd, Duffy (*rare*)	• Check the bilirubin level. • Check a direct Coombs test • Identify the antibody

CHAPTER 4

MEDICAL DISORDERS IN PREGNANCY

CARDIAC DISEASE

(For Cardiac Arrest, see p. 102; for Endocarditis Prophylaxis, see p. 110; for Anticoagulation for Valves, see p. 148.)

> Heart disease of varying types complicates less than 1% of all pregnancies but accounts for 9% of UK maternal deaths. While rheumatic heart disease remains a significant problem in the developing world, there are increasing numbers of fertile women in western countries who have had surgery for CHD as children. Maternal mortality is highest in those conditions where pulmonary blood flow cannot be increased to compensate for the increased demand during pregnancy, e.g. in those with pulmonary hypertension (particularly Eisenmenger syndrome, where maternal mortalities of 40–50% have been reported, Br J Obstet Gynaecol 1998:921).

Symptoms

Unfortunately many of the symptoms and signs usually considered indicative of heart disease occur commonly in normal pregnancy, and so making a clinical diagnosis is difficult:

- Breathlessness and syncopal episodes are present in 90% of normal pregnancies.
- Atrial and ventricular ectopic beats are common.
- Up to 96% of women may have an audible ejection systolic murmur. Refer to a cardiologist if >3/6, a thrill is present, or if there are any other suspicious features.
- 84% of women in pregnancy have a third heart sound.
- Murmurs over the right and left second intercostal space, which may be systolic or continuous, are common, and are due to mammary vessel blood flow.
- ECGs carried out in normal pregnancy may show depression of the ST segments, a Q wave in lead III and T wave flattening or inversion in V4, V5 and V6.
- A CXR may show slight cardiomegaly, increased pulmonary vascular markings and distension of pulmonary veins.

Antenatal management

A cardiologist should be involved at an early stage. If there are no haemodynamic problems (e.g. as with congenital mitral valve prolapse) then the prognosis is good and, after initial assessment, there is no need for cardiac follow-up. If there are significant potential haemodynamic problems, then consideration of pregnancy termination is an option (e.g. with Eisenmenger syndrome, primary pulmonary hypertension and pulmonary veno-occlusive disease). Heart failure should be treated medically (O_2, frusemide 20–50 mg slow IV, digoxin if AF or SVT). Open heart surgery should be avoided unless the mother's life is at risk. Anticoagulation is required with AF to prevent atrial clot forming and subsequent embolic problems.

Factors that increase the risk of heart failure should be avoided, e.g. infection, hypertension, anaemia and arrhythmias. All women with CHD should have a detailed USS of the fetus at 18–20 weeks, looking for cardiac anomalies (see 'Incidence of CHD in Offspring,' p. 12). If the maternal pO_2 is decreased, the fetus is at risk from asphyxia and IUGR and should be monitored with regular USS for growth, Doppler studies, CTGs and biophysical profiles.

SEVERE STRUCTURAL HEART DISEASE

There must be specialist involvement in delivery, particularly in those with prosthetic valves, aortic stenosis, severe mitral stenosis and those with pulmonary hypertension.

Management

- Heart disease in itself is not an indication for induction of labour.
- Labour should be conducted in a high dependency or ITU setting ±Swan–Ganz catheter monitoring (CVP monitoring may be misleading).
- Aim for a vaginal delivery, but avoid ↓BP, hypoxia or fluid overload. Epidural analgesia may be used, and is probably preferable to spinal block or GA (except where preloading is required to maintain output; e.g. HOCM, see below).
- Lie the patient on the left or right side, or in a semirecumbent position (to avoid aortocaval compression) with O_2 at 4–6 l/min and IV access.
- Endocarditis prophylaxis should be given if required (see below).
- The second stage should be kept short.
- Use Syntocinon 10 IU IV for the third stage rather than Syntometrine or ergometrine. Syntocinon 10 IU may be used even with cardiac failure.
- Particular care is required in the immediate postpartum period as there is an increased circulating volume following uterine constriction, which may lead to fluid overload and congestive failure (dilute any Syntocinon in a small volume).

Myocardial infarction

This is very rare in pregnancy but carries a high mortality, especially in the puerperium (25–50%). It may occur following coronary artery dissection in the absence of coronary atherosis. Creatinine kinase-MB is specific; lactic dehydrogenase may be misleading. Thrombolytic therapy is contraindicated during pregnancy as it may provoke placental haemorrhage. Those who have had an MI in pregnancy should be allowed to have a spontaneous delivery. A previous MI is not a contraindication to future pregnancies providing that cardiac function is satisfactory.

Cardiomyopathy

Puerperal cardiomyopathy. This is rare (<1:5000), carries a 25–50% mortality, and is associated with hypertension in pregnancy, multiple pregnancy, high multiparity and increased maternal age. It usually occurs in the puerperium (but may occur in late pregnancy) and presents with sudden onset of heart failure. There is a grossly dilated heart on echocardiography. Give frusemide, nitrates, ACE inhibitors and digoxin. Heparin reduces the risk of thromboembolism. Deliver (ideally vaginally) if it occurs antenatally. If there is good initial recovery, the long-term prognosis is good (although there is a risk of recurrence in future pregnancies).

Hypertrophic cardiomyopathy This is generally well tolerated in pregnancy unless there is severe outflow tract obstruction and heart failure. The risk of sudden death is probably not increased in pregnancy. Hypovolaemia should be avoided. Epidural anaesthesia should be used with caution only. Antiarrhythmic drugs may be required. β Blockers (e.g. sotalol) allow increased ventricular filling.

Aortic dissection

Pregnancy is associated with an increased risk of aortic dissection, particularly in women with heritable connective tissue disorders (e.g. Marfan's syndrome, Ehlers–Danlos syndrome) or in those with aortic coarctation. Those with an aortic root diameter >4 cm on ultrasound are at greatest risk, and risk may be increased further with hypertension ± a family history.

Dysryhthmias

Serious dysrhthymias are uncommon in pregnancy. Ventricular and atrial ectopic beats are common and are usually benign. Tachyarrhythmias are usually supraventricular. DC cardioversion and adenosine are safe in pregnancy.

ENDOCARDITIS PROPHYLAXIS

Strictly speaking, this is only required for patients with prosthetic valves or those who have had endocarditis. As treatment is simple, however, and the consequences of endocarditis grave, policies may vary in different areas:

- Give amoxycillin 1 g IM stat. and gentamicin 1.5 mg/kg (not to exceed 120 mg) IV stat. Thereafter, give amoxycillin 500 mg IM QID (PO, IV or IM) 6 hourly until the baby is born.
- If allergic to penicillin, vancomycin 1 g by slow IV infusion (over 2 hours) with gentamicin 1.5 mg/kg (not to exceed 120 mg) IV stat. is more appropriate.

CONNECTIVE TISSUE DISEASE

> Although these diseases are rare, they occur most commonly in women during their childbearing years and it is therefore relatively common to find them in association with pregnancy.

ANTIPHOSPHOLIPID ANTIBODY SYNDROME

Lupus anticoagulant and antiphospholipid antibodies are associated with recurrent miscarriage, arterial and venous thrombosis, IUGR, pre-eclampsia and thrombocytopenia. Of women with a history of recurrent miscarriage (3 or more consecutive pregnancy losses), 15% have persistently positive results for phospholipid antibodies and have a rate of fetal loss of 90% when untreated. There is now very good evidence that giving low-dose aspirin (75 mg/day) together with subcutaneous heparin (e.g. unfractionated subcutaneous heparin 5000 U BD or, and probably safer in terms of osteoporosis, Enoxaparin 40 mg/day SC) from the time of the first positive pregnancy test up until delivery results in a 71% incidence of live births (Br Med J 1997:253). The lupus anticoagulant is present in only 5–15% of patients with SLE, but commonly occurs in the absence of SLE.

SYSTEMIC LUPUS ERYTHEMATOSUS (SLE)

SLE occurs in 1:700 women aged 15–64 years. It is more common in non-white populations. The American Rheumatism Association diagnostic criteria require *four or more* of the following signs and symptoms:

1. butterfly rash,
2. discoid lupus,
3. photosensitivity,
4. oral or nasopharyngeal ulceration,
5. non-erosive arthritis involving two or more peripheral joints,
6. pleurisy or pericarditis,
7. proteinuria >0.5 mg/day,
8. psychosis,
9. convulsions

and *one* of the following:

1. haemolytic anaemia,
2. leucopenia or thrombocytopenia,
3. or immunological disorder (i.e. positive LE cell preparation, anti-DNA antibody, antinuclear antibody or chronically false-positive syphilis serology).

Effect of pregnancy on SLE

There is no effect on the long-term prognosis. There is probably an increased chance of flare-ups occurring in pregnancy (<20 weeks, ×3; 20–40 weeks, ×1.5; postpartum, ×6). Women should be discouraged from becoming pregnant during disease flare-ups in order to minimize fetal problems. Active SLE nephritis during pregnancy is associated with a significant maternal and perinatal mortality and in particular with a risk of pre-eclampsia.

Effect of SLE on pregnancy

SLE is associated with increased fetal loss rates from an increase in spontaneous abortions and preterm delivery. This is particularly so in those with raised anticardiolipin antibodies. In those pregnancies which reach term the perinatal mortality rate is similar to that of the general population. There is an increased incidence of pre-eclampsia and this may be difficult to differentiate from a disease flare-up as both are associated with hypertension and proteinuria. There is no increase in the rate of fetal abnormalities, although there is a risk of fetal CHB in association with the presence of anti-Ro and anti-La antibodies. Neonatal lupus may rarely occur, and is characterized by haemolytic anaemia, leucopenia, thrombocytopenia, discoid skin lesions, pericarditis and CHB.

Management of SLE in pregnancy *multidisciplinary < obst/phys | Combined Clinic*

- Check renal function with U&E and creatinine clearance.
- If lupus anticoagulant or anticardiolipin antibodies are present commence aspirin 75 mg/day until 36 weeks' gestation.
- If there is a previous history of thromboembolic disease, use SC low-dose heparin (e.g. 5000 U BD), or a low-molecular-weight heparin throughout pregnancy (see p. 147).
- If possible, maintain on simple analgesics (e.g. paracetamol) and try to avoid NSAIDs, particularly in the third trimester. There is now good data to show that chloroquine does not cause fetal retinal damage.
- Monitor disease activity with complement levels (reduced in active disease) and anti-DNA (increased in active disease).
- Flare-ups should be managed where possible with oral prednisolone (if already on oral prednisolone prior to labour continue with hydrocortisone 200 mg QID IV in labour). Steroids should be reduced very cautiously in the puerperium because of the risk of further disease flares. If steroids fail to control disease, then azathioprine appears to be relatively safe.
- Regular growth scans should be carried out, looking for IUGR as well as regular fetal monitoring with CTGs and biophysical profiles in the third trimester. There is no indication to deliver the fetus early unless there is evidence of fetal compromise, deteriorating maternal renal function or hypertension.
- CHB presents as prolonged fetal bradycardia on CTG and can lead to heart failure and non-immune hydrops. The baby may not cope with labour and CHB makes intrapartum fetal heart rate evaluation impossible. Elective caesarean section is appropriate.

○ Hypertension — 1st choice methyldopa → Nifedipine. Hydrallazine

RHEUMATOID ARTHRITIS

This usually improves during pregnancy although there is a risk of postpartum flare-up. There is no increased risk of fetal loss. There is, however, a small risk of CHB in association with anti-Ro or anti-La antibodies and there may be mechanical joint problems with delivery and anaesthesia. Treatment should be with simple paracetamol-based analgesics where possible. NSAIDs may be used with caution during the first and second trimesters but should be avoided if possible in the third trimester (where they are used, monitor the liquor volume). Prednisolone should be used to control severe disease if necessary. Sulphasalazine, azathioprine and chloroquine all appear to be relatively safe in pregnancy, but gold and penicillamine should be avoided.

SCLERODERMA

Scleroderma in its localized cutaneous form causes few problems in pregnancy. The diffuse cutaneous form which is associated with internal organ involvement carries a poor prognosis for mother and fetus, and pregnancy should be discouraged.

DIABETES

- **Impaired glucose tolerance:** an abnormality of the oral glucose tolerance test without the threshold for the diagnosis of diabetes being reached.
- **Gestational diabetes:** carbohydrate intolerance which arises during pregnancy and disappears after delivery (therefore a retrospective diagnosis).
- **Established diabetes:** diabetes which existed before pregnancy.

Screening in pregnancy with an oral GTT should be considered in all those with:

- significant glycosuria on two occasions antenatally, or one occasion before 16 weeks
- mother, father or siblings with diabetes,
- previous babies >90th centile for gestational age,
- diabetes in a previous pregnancy.

Some centres perform routine screening for diabetes on all women, since 30% of gestational diabetics have none of these features. This may be done by random blood sugar measurements with follow-up of abnormal levels (e.g. those with level ≥6 mmol/l two hours after food or ≥7 mmol/l at any time).

The normal fasting plasma glucose is < 5.8 mmol/l. For an oral GTT patients should fast overnight. Venous blood is taken for fasting blood glucose and a 75 g glucose drink is given. Further venous blood samples are taken after 1 hour and 2 hours. The WHO non-pregnant criteria are:

- *Diabetes:* fasting glucose >7.8 mmol/l and/or a 2 hour level of >11 mmol/l.
- *Impaired GT:* fasting glucose ≤7.8 mmol/l and a 2 hour level of ≤11 mmol/l but ≥8 mmol/l. (*Note:* In pregnancy, a 2 hour glucose of ≥9 mmol/l and ≤11 mmol/l may be more appropriate.) The significance of impaired GT is controversial. It is associated with obesity and one-third of those with impaired glucose tolerance go on to develop diabetes mellitus in the subsequent 25 years. There is no evidence that treatment is beneficial unless the results of the GTT suggest diabetes mellitus. It is reasonable to treat with diet in the first instance (unless the preprandial glucose is greater than 8 mmol/l) and to consider insulin if the preprandial level is still ≥6 mmol/l and/or the postprandial level is ≥8 mmol/l. The aim of insulin treatment is to keep the preprandial glucose level below 6 mmol/l.

Effects of pregnancy on diabetes

Insulin requirements may be static or decrease during the first trimester, increase during the second and third trimesters and may reduce slightly towards 40 weeks. Pregnancy exacerbates nephropathy, and in severe cases this may be an indication for termination. Pregnancy also exacerbates diabetic retinopathy and the eye should be monitored for proliferative retinopathy, and laser treatment given if required.

Nephropathy may be an indication for termination of pregnancy. Autonomic neuropathy may deteriorate, giving rise to postural hypotension and reduced hypoglycaemic awareness.

Effects of diabetes on pregnancy

The incidence of pre-eclampsia is increased. There is an increased incidence of maternal infection, particularly of the urinary tract, which may account in part for the increased incidence of preterm labour. Polyhydramnios may result in unstable lie and malpresentation, and may also lead to preterm labour.

↑ CS (30–60%)

Effects of diabetes on the fetus and neonate

There is an increased risk of spontaneous abortion and the perinatal mortality rate is 2–4 times that of the normal population. The incidence of congenital abnormalities is also 2–4 times that of the normal population, and accounts for 40% of perinatal mortality. The abnormalities are mainly cardiac defects, NTDs and renal anomalies. Caudal regression syndrome is very rare, but when it occurs it is usually associated with diabetes. The risk of congenital anomalies is increased if the maternal diabetic control is poor preconceptually and in the early stages of pregnancy, and also when there is evidence of maternal microvascular disease. Unexplained intrauterine fetal death (which is the other major contributor to perinatal mortality) may occur secondary to multiple factors, including chronic hypoxia, ketoacidosis, polycythaemia and lactic acidaemia. The macrosomic fetus may be more at risk because of the already increased O_2 demands.

Fetal macrosomia occurs in up to 40% of diabetic pregnancies. The risks are minimized if maternal blood glucose control is idealized and high postprandial blood glucose levels avoided. Labour and delivery may be complicated by dystocia and, in particular, shoulder dystocia. IUGR occurs in 20% of diabetic pregnancies, particularly in association with pre-eclampsia and maternal vascular disease. Fetal hypertrophic cardiomyopathy characterized by a thick intraventricular septum and left ventricular outflow obstruction is common in diabetic pregnancy and may cause fetal death. It is reversible over a few weeks if the infant survives.

Neonates may have hypoglycaemia, hypocalcaemia, hypomagnesaemia and polycythaemia. There is also an increased incidence of respiratory distress syndrome.

Management of diabetes in pregnancy

At pre-pregnancy counselling advice should be given about good diabetic control, diet, smoking and folate supplements. Diagnose and treat retinopathy. Change those on oral hypoglycaemics to insulin. If possible, pregnancy management should be in a combined obstetric/diabetic clinic. Visits are often fortnightly. Blood glucose should be measured several times a day at home, aiming for tight control (e.g. with preprandial levels <5 mmol/l and 1–2 hour postprandial levels of <7.5 mmol/l). HbA1 should be checked monthly, aiming for <8%.

Insulin is commonly given in a soluble form preprandially three times daily, with an intermediate insulin overnight. Ketoacidosis should be avoided, as it is associated with a significant perinatal mortality.

Maternal renal function, weight, BP and optic fundi should be checked at each visit. Offer serum screening and a detailed scan at 16–18 weeks to detect fetal anomalies. Examine the abdomen for polyhydramnios, macrosomia or IUGR (particularly common if microvascular disease is present) and consider serial growth scans (unproven value). In the third trimester regular assessments of fetal well-being (CTG or biophysical profile) may be carried out, but note that the CTG may be abnormal when plasma glucose is elevated or reduced. Also note that the use of liquor to assess fetal well-being may be flawed in diabetes as there is an increased possibility of polyhydramnios.

With regard to delivery, each case should be considered separately. There is no need for intervention before 40 weeks if there is no evidence of complications, and there is no indication for elective caesarean section on the basis of diabetes alone. If preterm labour occurs, steroids should be given as for the non-diabetic patient, but there may be marked deterioration in diabetic control (consider using an insulin IV infusion). β-Sympathomimetics may cause hyperglycaemia.

Contraception

The COC pill is not recommended in diabetics as there is an increased risk of thromboembolism and glucose tolerance is adversely affected. The progestogen only pill is a reasonable alternative. The IUCD may be used.

DIABETES AND DELIVERY

There are numerous different IV regimens. Some favour 'single infusions' (e.g. 10% dextrose with 10 mmol KCl and 10 U of Actrapid). A possible 'separate infusions' regimen is outlined below. Always involve a diabetic physician.

It is important to differentiate those with IDDM from those with gestational diabetes. Those with IDDM will need insulin during delivery, whereas those with gestational diabetes, even if they have been on large doses of insulin during pregnancy, are most unlikely to need insulin during labour and only rarely postpartum. It is most important to ensure that IDDM patients always have some insulin being infused. Discontinuing the infusion may result in ketosis within approximately 1–2 hours. In the immediate postpartum period most IDDM patients require no insulin, and regular BMs are essential with a view to re-establishing a subcutaneous regimen. Dextrose (5%) or normal saline may be used for IV fluid replacement. It is not necessary to use 5% dextrose solely; there is a risk of water overload and gluconeogenesis will continue in the fasting state anyway.

Caesarean section

This can be divided into six groups, as below.

Management

For those requiring insulin, make up an IV solution by adding 50 U of Actrapid insulin to 50 ml of normal saline (1 ml = 1 U) and infuse according to the sliding scale in Table 4.1. Fluids can be given entirely independently of this.

TABLE 4.1 Sliding scale for insulin administration by IV infusion

BM (mmol/l) every 2 h	Rate of infusion (ml/h)
>16	4
13–15.9	3
10–12.9	2
6.5–9.9	1
<6.5	0.5

IDDM patients undergoing elective caesarean section Give the normal insulin on the night before the operation (although consider reducing the intermediate- or long-acting insulin). On the morning of the operation, omit the morning insulin, check U&E and glucose and insert an IV cannula. Infuse fluids and insulin as in Table 4.1.

Gestational diabetics who have required no insulin during pregnancy for elective caesarean section Perform BMs 4-hourly, although it is expected that all values will be <10 mmol/l. Give IV fluids as required. If BM levels are consistently above 10 mmol/l then commence insulin as above, stopping it on delivery of the placenta.

Gestational diabetics who have required insulin in pregnancy for elective caesarian section Give the usual evening insulin. Check the U&E and glucose on the morning of the operation and establish IV access. Monitor BMs 2-hourly and commence insulin as in Table 4.1 if the BMs are >10 mmol/l. Stop any infusion after the delivery.

IDDM patients undergoing emergency caesarean section Check the U&E and glucose. Start an IV infusion of 5% dextrose 500 ml over 4 hours and run insulin through a separate infusion as in Table 4.1. Postdelivery insulin requirements frequently drop, so switch the infusion off and monitor the BMs every 2 hours. Recommence the infusion if the BM is >10 mmol/l. Continue IV fluids, adding potassium to the bags if required. Discontinue the insulin infusion 30 minutes after the first SC insulin injection to ensure an adequate overlap.

Gestational diabetics who have required no insulin during pregnancy undergoing emergency caesarean section No specific measures are required and insulin therapy is unlikely to be needed. Carry out BM testing every 4 hours and commence an insulin infusion if BMs are >10 mmol/l. IV fluids may be given as required. Stop any infusion after the delivery.

Gestational diabetics who have required insulin in pregnancy undergoing emergency caesarean section Check the preoperative U&E and glucose. Establish IV access and give dextrose 500 ml over 4 hours. Check BMs 2-hourly and give insulin if the BM is >10 mmol/l. Stop any infusion after the delivery.

Vaginal delivery

Management

For all those who have required insulin antenatally:

- It is possible to manage patients with their normal SC insulin and oral intake in labour, providing labour is progressing normally.
- If the patient needs to fast, commence an IV infusion with 500 ml 10% dextrose at a *constant* rate of 100 ml/h. Make up an IV solution by adding 50 U of Actrapid insulin to 50 ml of normal saline (1 ml = 1 U) and infuse according to the sliding scale in Table 4.1, checking the BMs on an hourly basis.

- Stop the infusion immediately postdelivery, continuing hourly BMs for the first 4 hours. Recommence SC insulin (at previous non-pregnant dose) when the BM is >10 mmol/l.

DIABETIC KETOACIDOSIS

There is a high fetal loss rate due to fetal hypoxia from keto- and lactic acidosis. It occurs most commonly with IDDM, but may rarely occur with gestational diabetes, especially if β-agonists are used. The aim is to restore intravascular volume, lower the glucose, monitor electrolyte status and correct the acid–base balance.

Remember
Always involve a diabetic physician.

Investigations

- BM stix, glucose and urinalysis for ketones.
- FBC, U&E, creatinine, glucose, ABGs and G&S.
- Fetal assessment with CTG and consideration of delivery depending on gestation and fetal well-being. Delivery of a compromised fetus should be delayed until the mother is metabolically stable.
- Search for a cause: blood cultures, HVS, MSU and sputum for bacteriology, CXR, ECG.

Management

Establish IV access and give 1000 ml of 0.9% saline and 6 U Actrapid IV stat. while awaiting the blood results.

- If Na^+ >155 mmol/l, give 0.45% saline at 1000 ml/h until the Na^+ is <155 mmol/l. If the Na^+ is <155 mmol/l, continue with 0.9% saline at 125 ml/h for 4 hours.
- Set up a continuous insulin infusion (after stat. dose as above). Add 5 U of Actrapid to 50 ml normal saline and run it at 5 U/h until the glucose is <14 mmol/l (increase to 10 U/h if the glucose is not <25% in 2 hours). Thereafter give 500 ml of 10% dextrose with 10 mmol KCl in each bag at 100 ml/h and Actrapid as below:
  — if glucose >12 mmol/l, add 14 U to each bag,
  — if glucose 7–12 mmol/l, add 10 U to each bag,
  — if glucose <7 mmol/l, add 6 U to each bag.
- Add KCl to each bag depending on the K^+ result (5 ml of 15% KCl = 10 mmol), re-checking the level initially every 1–2 hours:
  — K^+ <3.0 mmol/l, 40 mmol in each bag,

— K^+ 3.0–4.0 mmol/l, 20 mmol in each bag,

— K^+ 4.0–5.0 mmol/l, 10 mmol in each bag,

— K^+ >5.0 mmol/l, give no K^+.

- If >6.5 mmol/l, there may be tented T waves with a prolonged QRS and there is a risk of arrhythmias. Give 50 ml of 50% dextrose IV and 10 U Actrapid IV. If >8.0 mmol/l, also give 10 ml 10% calcium gluconate slow IV (for cardioprotective effect).
- If the pH is <7.10 on ABG give 40 mmol (i.e. 40 ml) of 8.4% $NaHCO_3$ slow IV.

HYPOGLYCAEMIA

The blood glucose is <2.2 mmol/l, although symptoms may occur before this level.

- If conscious, give sweet tea, milk or dextrose tablets or Hypostop.
- If unconscious:
    - 1 mg (1 vial) of glucagon IM or SC (should be available at home),
    - if no response, give 20–50 ml of 50% dextrose IV (irritates the vein),
    - if there is no glucagon and a vein cannot be found, give 50 ml of 50% dextrose via a nasogastric tube.
- Consider the cause.
- Do not omit the next dose of insulin.

DRUG MISUSE

> The prevalence of drug misuse is on the increase, particularly in women of childbearing age. Serious problem misuse (especially IV) and poly-drug misuse is associated with socio-economic deprivation and an increase in obstetric complications including miscarriage, APH, IUGR, IUD and preterm labour. Care must usually be directed firmly towards social factors before any impact on obstetric problems can be achieved. Pregnancy may provide a window of opportunity to provide real help, often breaking a cycle of poor parenting, which leads in turn to further problems in the next generation.

History should cover the following:

- Type of drug:
    - street drugs (e.g. heroin, amphetamines),
    - pharmacological preparations (usually illicit and/or prescribed) (e.g. benzodiazepines, buprenorphine and analgesics (particularly DF 118 and other codeine compounds),
    - prescribed preparations (usually methadone).

- Pattern of use, dose, route, frequency and method of financing supply.
- Social support, the other children, partner, family, friends, social work involvement, clothing, food, shelter and transport.
- Impending legal problems.
- Risks of infection, including HIV, hepatitis B/C counselling ± testing (see p. 135).
- Domestic abuse is a common occurrence with all groups of pregnant women, and all women should be asked about this (surprisingly, it is not any more common in association with socio-economic deprivation). Female drug misuse is often a consequence, rather than a cause, of violence.

The women may have poor self esteem following a lack of trusting relationships, a lack of a positive body image and concerns about their own abilities to be a parent.

Management

Social factors Illegal drugs are expensive and addicts are often forced into theft (and therefore problems with the police and courts) or prostitution (with its risks of violence and sexually transmitted diseases, including HIV). In addition, the lifestyle may be erratic and pregnancy outcome is compounded by various additional nutritional and social factors. Attendance for antenatal care may often compete with more immediate problems (e.g. seeing the social worker, lawyer, or getting money/drugs), but if such care can be delivered locally with truly flexible access and be combined with confidentiality, non-judgmental consistency, access to social workers and legal aid, then fuller and more holistic care can be achieved.

Opiate/opioid users For these women, consider transfer to methadone (this is metabolized more slowly than opiates/opioids, and therefore remains at more stable levels and there is less risk of fetal distress and preterm labour associated with sudden withdrawals or fluctuations in serum opiate levels). Those stabilized on methadone alone probably have a lower neonatal mortality than those still taking heroin (Addiction 1998:93). There may also be improved prenatal attendance. There is still no appropriate substitution therapy for other commonly abused drugs.

Detoxification There are theoretical fetal risks from very rapid opiate/opioid detoxification, but in practice the true fetal risks from even 'cold turkey' detoxification are relatively small. It has been suggested that the risks of detoxification (whether rapid or gradual) may be higher in the first and third trimesters, but practical experience does not bear this out. The goal should be to reduce drug use to a level compatible with stability (e.g. with methadone), not necessarily aiming for abstinence. It may be more acceptable for a mother taking a moderate dose of methadone to top up with very small amounts of a similar non-infected substance (e.g. smoking heroin) rather than increasing methadone doses to very high levels in a futile attempt to achieve total abstinence from illicit drugs. In women who attempt unrealistic reductions in methadone and do top up with other drugs, the dose of methadone should be increased. Topping up with benzodiazepines is particularly inadvisable. Patients undergoing rapid detoxification should ideally be managed on an obstetric unit, or at least under the close supervision of an obstetrician.

Neonatal complications

The effects of "recreational" drugs on the fetus are summarized in Table 4.2. There is an increased incidence of low birthweight due to IUGR ± preterm delivery and SIDS. Opiate/opioid use is associated with an increased incidence of meconium aspiration. Withdrawal is particularly associated with opiates/opioids and benzodiazepines, and is worse if these drugs have been used together. Severity is dose related and timing depends on the rate of

TABLE 4.2   Fetal effects of drugs

Drug	Effect on fetus
Alcohol	There is no clear dose relationship. Fetal alcohol syndrome (IUGR, microcephaly, craniofacial abnormalities and mental retardation) is rare. Consumption of even small amounts of alcohol has been associated with a reduction in birthweight and intellectual impairment
Amphetamines	There is no good evidence of fetal abnormality. Fetal thrombocytopenia is very rare
Benzodiazepines	Neonatal withdrawal occurs at levels associated with abuse, even after quite brief use. 'Floppy infant syndrome' may occur if high doses have been given to a non-abusing mother in the 15 hours prior to delivery
Ecstasy	No increased risk has been demonstrated
Cannabis (hash, marihuana)	There have been no demonstrable teratogenic effects, but there is an association (? indirect) with IUGR
Opiates/opioids (e.g. heroin, methadone, DF 118, buprenorphine)	Methadone and heroin are associated with IUGR, and heroin is also associated with amenorrhoea (± anovulation) and preterm labour. Buprenorphine and DF 118 probably have similar associations to heroin, but with DF 118 there is increased severity of withdrawal
Cocaine and crack	Cocaine has been associated (rarely) with GU, limb/body and brain abnormalities (probably due to vasoconstrictive vascular accidents). There is an increased risk of abruption, PROM and possibly IUGR and SIDS
Nicotine	There is an association with IUGR, preterm labour, perinatal death and delayed development. Tobacco use, if heavy, may lead to neonatal withdrawals
LSD	No increased risk has been demonstrated

drug metabolism (e.g. heroin and morphine are metabolized rapidly) and signs usually develop within 1 day, whereas methadone is metabolized more slowly and signs usually occur at 3–5 days. Babies are classically hungry, but feed ineffectually. There is CNS hyperexcitability (increased reflexes and tremor), GI dysfunction (finger sucking, regurgitation, diarrhoea) and respiratory distress. Treatment options include replacement (e.g. with methadone or Oramorph) for those who have been taking opiates/opioids. Replacement is not appropriate for benzodiazepine withdrawals. The severity of withdrawal symptoms is reduced by breast-feeding.

EPILEPSY AND OTHER NEUROLOGICAL DISORDERS

Assume that a seizure during pregnancy is eclampsia until proven otherwise. Around a third of epileptics have an increase in seizure frequency independent of the effects of medication, particularly those with secondary generalized or complex partial seizures. The fall in anticonvulsant levels due to dilution, reduced absorption, reduced compliance and increased drug metabolism is partially compensated for by reduced protein binding (and therefore an increase in the level of free drug). There is an increased incidence in fetal anomaly in epileptics irrespective of the effects of drugs (3–4% vs 2% in the general population), possibly due to a combination of hypoxic and genetic factors. For those on anticonvulsants, the incidence of anomaly is ≈6%, (see p. 35). Single-drug regimens are less teratogenic than multidrug therapy.

EPILEPSY

Management

Pre-pregnancy counselling This is advised. Fertility is not impaired. Attempt to achieve seizure control with a single-drug regime or, if seizure free for 2–3 years, consider drug withdrawal (this may have implications for the patient's work ± driving licence). Give pre-conception folate supplements 5 mg/day PO (anticonvulsants lead to a reduction in serum folate).

During pregnancy Continue folate supplementation until at least 12 weeks. Adjust anticonvulsant doses on clinical grounds (monitoring of plasma levels is usually not necessary, but can occasionally be useful to check compliance and exclude toxicity – 'free' drug levels rather than 'total' drug levels are ideal). If the level is low and the seizure frequency low, it may be acceptable not to increase the dose. In those taking anticonvulsants, it should be emphasized that there are fetal risks from the anticonvulsant medication as well as from not taking the drugs (from increased fit frequency). Offer aneuploidy screening as usual, but arrange a detailed fetal anomaly scan at 18–22 weeks (looking for neural tube, cardiac and craniofacial abnormalities as well as diaphragmatic herniae). For women on enzyme inducing anticonvulsants (see below), give vitamin K 20 mg/day PO from 36 weeks (anticonvulsants are vitamin K antagonists and increase the risk of haemorrhagic disease of the newborn). The baby should be given vitamin K 1 mg IM stat. at birth and the paediatrician alerted to the possibilities of anticonvulsant drug withdrawal. Most fits in pregnancy will be self-limiting, but if prolonged give Diazemuls 10 mg IV or diazepam 10 mg PR. If still continuing, give phenytoin by infusion and, if very prolonged, consider ventilation.

Postnatally The mother may breast-feed safely (drugs pass into the milk but are of little clinical significance). Advise about safe and suitable settings for feeding, bathing, etc. (Useful UK contacts can be found through The Joint Epilepsy Council, tel. 0113 243 9393.) Carbamazepine, phenytoin, primidone and phenobarbitone induce liver enzymes, reducing the effectiveness of the standard dose COCs. Therefore, consider a 50 μg preparation (e.g. Ovran) or give $2 \times 25/30$ μg pills and reduce the number of pill-free intervals by running three packets together.

OTHER NEUROLOGICAL DISORDERS

(See also: Prolactinoma, p. 184; Carpal Tunnel Syndrome, p. 48.)

Migraine
This generally improves in pregnancy. Paracetamol and antiemetics for treatment with β-blockers as prophylaxis are considered relatively safe. Focal migraine is associated with an increased risk of stroke during pregnancy and patients should therefore commence prophylactic treatment.

Cerebrovascular disease
This is rare. Subarachnoid haemorrhage is nearly always secondary to an aneurysm (>25 years old, >30 weeks pregnant) or AV malformation (<20 years old, 15–20 weeks pregnant). Those who have a previously clipped aneurysm should be allowed to labour, although it is reasonable not to allow a prolonged second stage.

Paraplegia
Assess renal function antenatally and check for urinary infection regularly. If the lesion is above T10, labour will be painless. If above T6, there is a risk of intrapartum autonomic hyperreflexia (leading to severe hypertension);

therefore insert an epidural or give antihypertensives. Avoid bladder distension. Forceps are often required, caesarean section rarely so.

Multiple sclerosis
The risk of relapse during pregnancy is reduced, but is increased for 6 months postpartum, so that the overall relapse rate is the same as for the non-pregnant patient.

GASTROINTESTINAL DISORDERS

Peptic ulceration
Ulcers are rare in pregnancy but, when present, tend to improve. If ulcer symptoms occur, first-line treatment is with simple antacid/alginate compounds. If not resolving then use ranitidine 300 mg/day PO. Those with problematic recurrent ulcers should also take ranitidine. Endoscopy is the investigation of choice if necessary.

Inflammatory bowel disease (IBD)
Fetal loss rate is similar to that of the normal population, providing that the disease is not active at the start of pregnancy. Flare-ups of disease occur most commonly in the first trimester. There is no evidence of any fetal problems with prednisolone or sulphasalazine and these should be continued at the minimum dose necessary. Avoid constipation. Give folic acid supplements.

Acute episodes of IBD present with abdominal pain, diarrhoea and passage of blood and mucus PR. Patients should be admitted and the fluid and electrolyte balance checked. Stool samples should be sent for culture to exclude gastroenteritis. Treatment is with topical steroid enemas, oral sulphasalazine 1 g BD and prednisolone 10–20 mg/day. If the patient deteriorates, consider the possibility of intestinal perforation or toxic megacolon. Colostomies and ileostomies may become temporarily obstructed during pregnancy. Vaginal deliveries are preferable to caesarean section (as there is a risk of adhesions from previous surgery), although care is needed with operative vaginal deliveries if the disease involves the perineum. Although sulphasalazine crosses into breast milk there is no evidence of any neonatal problems.

Coeliac disease
Presentation may occur in pregnancy with non-specific GI symptoms, anaemia and weight loss. Diagnosis is by duodenal biopsy via endoscopy. Treat with a gluten-free diet and vitamin supplementation. Patients with known coeliac disease should be encouraged to comply with a strict gluten-free diet. Iron and folate supplements are recommended. The prognosis for the mother and fetus is good.

HEPATIC DISORDERS

> A history of a prodromal illness, overseas travel or high-risk group for blood-borne illness may suggest viral hepatitis. Itch is suggestive of cholestasis. Abdominal pain is associated with gallstones, HELLP syndrome and acute fatty liver. Clinical signs are often unhelpful in diagnosis. Check the U&E, urate, LFTs, blood glucose, platelets and coagulation screen. Take blood for hepatitis serology. Upper abdominal USS may show obstruction or fat infiltration. Alkaline phosphatase increases in pregnancy (1.5–2 times normal).

LIVER DISORDERS SPECIFIC TO PREGNANCY

Hyperemesis gravidarum

If severe, this may be associated with abnormal LFTs (see p. 46).

Intrahepatic cholestasis of pregnancy

Incidence 1:1000 pregnancies. This is a familial condition characterized by mild jaundice. It usually presents after 30 weeks' gestation possibly due to a genetic predisposition to the cholestatic effect of oestrogens. There is a family history in up to 50% of cases. Pruritus is generally severe, affecting the limbs and trunk. There is a moderate (less than threefold) increase in transaminases and a raised alkaline phosphatase (above normal pregnancy values). Bilirubin is usually <100 μmol/l, and there may be pale stools and dark urine. Serum total bile acid concentration is increased early in the disease and may be the optimum marker (not available in most UK laboratories).

There are no serious long-term maternal risks but there is a risk of preterm labour, fetal distress and intrauterine fetal death. The fetus must be monitored closely and there is growing evidence that delivery at 37–38 weeks is appropriate. Itch is difficult to control, but chlorpheniramine 4 mg QID PO may be helpful. Give vitamin K 10 mg/day PO to the mother predelivery. Cholestyramine can be given, but is unpleasant to take, is often unsuccessful at relieving symptoms and may exacerbate vitamin K deficiency. More recently, ursodeoxycholic acid has been used with success and, although unlicensed in pregnancy, there have been no adverse fetal side-effects. If LFTs do not return to normal after delivery, then exclude primary biliary cirrhosis. The COC pill is contraindicated.

HELLP syndrome

See page 133.

Acute fatty liver of pregnancy (Curr Opinion Nephrol 1994:436)

Incidence 1:10 000 pregnancies. This very rare condition carries a high maternal and fetal mortality and may progress rapidly to hepatic failure.

It usually presents with vomiting in the third trimester associated with malaise and abdominal pain. This is followed by jaundice, thirst and alteration in consciousness level. LFTs are elevated, urate is very high and there is often profound hypoglycaemia. There may be hypertension and proteinuria. Once the diagnosis is made, correct any coagulopathy, hypoglycaemia and fluid imbalance. Monitor the fetus continuously and prepare for delivery, usually by caesarean section. Following delivery there is a risk of PPH and liver dysfunction may be prolonged. Hepatic encephalopathy may develop and liver transplant is occasionally necessary. If the patient recovers, there is no long-term liver impairment.

OTHER LIVER DISORDERS

Viral hepatitis
This is the commonest cause of abnormal LFTs in pregnancy. Check hepatitis A, B and C titres, as well as for CMV and toxoplasmosis (see p. 135).

Cholelithiasis
Asymptomatic gallstones do not require treatment. Cholecystitis should be managed conservatively with analgesia, bed rest, IV fluids and broad-spectrum IV antibiotics. Check amylase to exclude pancreatitis. Obstruction of the bile duct requires surgical treatment.

Cirrhosis
In severe disease there is usually amenorrhoea. If pregnancy occurs, and the disease is well compensated, there is usually no long-term effect on hepatic function. The main risk is from bleeding oesophageal varices. During pregnancy, patients should rest and take a high-carbohydrate, low-protein diet. Constipation should be avoided. Vaginal delivery is safe, but avoid a prolonged second stage. Sedative drugs should be used with caution as they may precipitate encephalopathy.

Chronic active hepatitis
This is usually associated with amenorrhoea. Pregnancy does not usually have any long-term effect on liver function. Obstetric complications are common and fetal loss rate is high. Immunosuppressant therapy with prednisolone and azathioprine should be continued in those with autoimmune disease.

Primary biliary cirrhosis
This is variable in severity. The prognosis for mother and fetus is good in mild disease. It may present during pregnancy for the first time in a similar way to intrahepatic cholestasis of pregnancy.

Acute pancreatitis

This may be more severe in pregnancy and the fetal loss rate is ≈10%. Serum amylase is markedly elevated. Treatment is with fasting, bed rest, IV fluids, oxygen and correction of any glucose and electrolyte balance (including calcium and magnesium).

Dewhurst +/ Nelsonpuercy

HYPERTENSION

> Hypertension in pregnancy is defined as a diastolic BP >110 mmHg on any one occasion or >90 mmHg on two occasions ≥4 hours apart (ISSHP classification). Severe hypertension is a single diastolic BP >120 mmHg on any one occasion or >110 mmHg on two occasions ≥4 hours apart. In normal pregnancy the BP will fall during the first trimester, reaching a nadir in the second trimester and rising slightly again during the third trimester. Measure in the sitting position with an appropriate size of cuff. Although controversial, it is suggested that the phase IV Korotkoff sound (i.e. 'muffling' rather than 'disappearance') should be taken when reading the diastolic pressure.

Raised BP at booking (e.g. <16 weeks) is usually due to chronic hypertension (usually essential hypertension and only rarely renal disease or phaeochromocytoma). Gestational hypertension and pre-eclampsia (hypertension and proteinuria) only very rarely occur <20 weeks (with the exception of trophoblastic disease). Check FBC, U&E and urine dipstix, and consider renal USS and separate 24-hour urine collections for creatinine clearance and urinary catecholamines.

ESSENTIAL HYPERTENSION

This is commoner in older women and the prognosis overall is good. The *16-18 %* main risk is from superimposed pre-eclampsia (which is more common with pre-existing essential hypertension). The hypertension itself is rarely of significance, although there might be a slightly increased risk of abruption. *1-9 %* Those women, who are already taking antihypertensive drugs, and who have mild to moderate hypertension (140/90–170/110 mmHg), may be able to discontinue the medication in pregnancy. Those with more severe hypertension should continue.

Treatment

Methyldopa This is the treatment of choice as it has a proven safety record (250–750 mg QID PO).

β **Blockers** Labetalol can be used, but there may be an adverse effect on fetal growth if used over a prolonged period of time (100 mg TID to 400 mg QID PO).

Nifedipine This can be used, and is particularly useful as a second-line agent where there is superimposed pre-eclampsia (10–40 mg BD PO).

Diuretics These should be avoided because of the relatively reduced intravascular fluid volume, particularly if there is any evidence of the development of pre-eclampsia.

ACE inhibitors These are contraindicated throughout pregnancy because of adverse effects on the fetal renal system, but are useful agents in the puerperium.

GESTATIONAL HYPERTENSION AND PRE-ECLAMPSIA

- Gestational hypertension: see definitions above, but note that some authorities also consider an incremental diastolic rise of >25 mmHg above booking to be significant.
- Gestational proteinuria:
  — either ≥300 mg/24 h,
  — or two clean-catch specimens at least 4 hours apart with ≥++ protein, or ≥+ if the urine SG is <1.030 (i.e. dilute) and the pH is <8 (higher false positive rates with alkaline urine; overall false positive rate with dipstick ≈ 10%)

Pre-eclampsia is a multisystem disorder of unknown aetiology peculiar to pregnancy and characterized by hypertension, proteinuria and, often, fluid retention. There is reduced maternal plasma volume and increased vascular permeability, some degree of intravascular coagulopathy (may lead to DIC), glomerular damage (proteinuria), liver dysfunction (see HELLP syndrome, below), cardiac failure, pulmonary oedema, CNS problems (eclampsia, haemorrhage) and adverse fetal effects. It is an extremely variable and unpredictable condition, and progression is often more rapid the earlier in pregnancy it occurs. The purpose of antenatal screening is to prevent both the maternal complications (cerebral injury, multisystem failure) and fetal complications (IUGR, intrauterine death, abruption) of severe disease by timely delivery of the baby. Treatment of the mother with antihypertensives masks the sign of hypertension but does not alter the course of the disease, although it may allow prolongation of the pregnancy and thereby improve fetal outcome.

Investigations → Ch. of Preeclampsia, preceed 1–2 week to preeclampsia level correlati c severity & mip. in prognosis

- Urate: this increases as pregnancy advances. (*Note:* levels may be higher in the obese.) The mean level is:
  — 232 μmol/l at 28 weeks,
  — 269 μmol/l at 36 weeks.
- Platelets: these fall as the disease progresses, although there is a small physiological fall in platelets towards the end of pregnancy. The rate of fall of platelets is important as well as the absolute level itself.

Management of gestational hypertension → Refer Dewhurst
The following may be used as guidelines:

- If the BP is found to be elevated at an antenatal visit, recheck after 10–20 minutes. If settled, no further action is required.
- If the BP is elevated on ≥2 occasions ≥4 hours apart, appraise fetal size clinically, enquire about maternal well-being and advise to present if unwell or if frontal headache or epigastric pain. Check serum urate, U&E, FBC and platelets. Arrange twice-weekly BP recording and urine 'dipstix' measurement.
- If there are abnormal blood results, or diastolic BP is >100 mmHg, or has risen from booking by >25 mmHg, or there is clinical suspicion of IUGR, or poor fetal or maternal well-being, arrange for a CTG and USS assessment of fetal size and liquor volume. Also, arrange BP recording and 'dipstix' three times weekly, with at least weekly serum urate, U&E, FBC and platelets.

It is important to consider the overall picture rather than make decisions on the basis of a single factor. It is appropriate to admit the mother if there are symptoms or if there is significant proteinuria or severe hypertension. More intensive monitoring is possible, oral antihypertensives may be considered and plans can be made for delivery.

The decision to deliver and the method of delivery are dependent on many of the above factors and must be tailored to each individual patient. There are probably advantages to conservative management <34 weeks if BP, laboratory values and fetal parameters are stable (Obstet Gynecol 1990;76: 1070, Am J Obstet Gynecol 1994:818). An epidural is probably contraindicated if platelets are <100 × 10^9/l (or ? <50 × 10^9/l). Ergometrine (including syntometrine) should not be used for the third stage (give Syntocinon 10 U IM or IV stat. instead).

It has been suggested that low-dose aspirin taken from early pregnancy (<17 weeks and probably from the first trimester) may reduce the incidence of IUGR or perinatal mortality in those with previous disease. Studies found that it may be of benefit in high-risk situations and that it is safe (Lancet 1994;343:619). Haemorrhage is not a problem, even though there is a moderate prolongation of bleeding time.

Severe pre-eclampsia/eclampsia

Eclampsia is said to have occurred when there has been a convulsion. The UK national incidence is 4.9/10 000 pregnancies, with 38% occurring antepartum, 18% intrapartum and 44% postnatal. Of these 38% occur before proteinuria and hypertension have been documented. The mortality is 1.8%, with a neonatal death rate of 34/1000 (Br Med J 1994:1395). See the definition of severe hypertension (above), but symptoms, or the presence of a coagulopathy, also suggest severe disease.

Management of eclampsia

- Turn on side to avoid aortocaval compression.
- Insert an airway and give high-flow O_2 (e.g. 6 l/min).
- Give 4 g $MgSO_4$ over 10–15 minutes (details below).
- Consider urgent delivery if the fit has occurred antenatally.
- Set up a 1 g/h IV infusion of $MgSO_4$ (as below) and manage as for severe pre-eclampsia.
- Consider paralysis and ventilation if the fits are prolonged or recurrent.

Management of severe pre-eclampsia and ongoing eclampsia

The aim is to reduce diastolic BP to <100 mmHg, prevent pulmonary oedema, prevent convulsions and maintain the urine output.

- Gain initial IV access.
- Check the U&E, LFTs, albumin, urate, Hb, H'CRIT, platelets and clotting.
- Perform a CTG for fetal assessment.
- Give consideration to the method and timing of delivery.
- Catheterize.
- Measure hourly urine volumes.
- Control BP with hypotensive therapy.
- The aim is to reduce the BP slowly. Also consider giving labetolol, hydralazine (or nifedipine) as below.

Labetolol (Trandate) This comes as ampoules of 100 mg in 20 ml.

- Give an initial bolus: 50 mg (10 ml) slowly IV over 2–5 min.
- Then set up an infusion: add the ampoules undiluted to a syringe driver (5 mg/ml) starting at 4 ml/h, doubling every 30 min to a maximum of 32 ml/h (160 mg/h).

Side-effects If used along with hydralazine there may be profound hypotension. Continuous BP monitoring is required and, if the patient becomes symptomatically hypotensive, give atropine 600 µg IV stat. Caution is required with asthma, and labetolol is contraindicated in those with AV block.

Hydralazine (Apresoline) This comes as ampoules containing 20 mg in powder form. Dissolve in 1 ml of water and make up to 20 ml with normal saline.

- Give a bolus: 5–10 mg slowly over at least 2 minutes.
- Then start an infusion: make this up as 80 µg/ml (i.e. 40 mg hydralazine to 500 ml Hartmann's solution). Start at 30 ml/h (40 µg/min), increasing by 30 ml/h every 30 min to 120 ml/h (160 µg/min) or until the BP is controlled. Wean off by reducing by 30 ml/h every 30 min.

Side-effects Tachycardia and severe headache (therefore there may be confusion with eclamptic symptoms). Its use along with a β blocker may cause profound hypotension. Continuous BP monitoring is required, and if the patient becomes hypotensive give atropine 600 µg IV stat.

Nifedipine Give a 5–10 mg capsule sublingually, and repeat if required, to a maximum of 40 mg. (*Caution:* with $MgSO_4$ nifedipine may lead to increased BP.)

Side-effects Headache (therefore it may be confused with eclamptic symptoms).

Anticonvulsant therapy

There is now very good evidence supporting the use of anticonvulsants in established eclampsia, and magnesium sulphate is known to be significantly more effective than phenytoin or diazepam in preventing further convulsions (Lancet 1995;345:1455). Although the use of $MgSO_4$ in severe pre-eclampsia has been shown to be effective in preventing eclampsia (Br J Obstet Gynaecol 1998:300), treatment is not without risk. The results from further trials are expected (including the MAGPIE trial, Oxford).

Magnesium sulphate (CI with myasthenia gravis).

- Take one 20 ml vial of 20% $MgSO_4$ (= 4 g) and infuse intravenously over 10–15 min. If the patient is anuric, do not administer further $MgSO_4$ until urine is produced. Providing there is urine production, infuse 1 g/h (5 ml/h) via a syringe pump, continuing for 24 h after the last fit.
- If further convulsions occur, give a further 2 g (or 4 g if the body weight is >70 kg) IV over 5 min.

Measure the respiratory rate and confirm that the patellar reflex is present (or forearm reflex in a patient with an epidural) every 15 minutes. If it is not possible to check these on such a frequent basis, $MgSO_4$ levels may be checked at 1 and 4 hours after commencement of treatment, and 6 hourly thereafter, aiming for 2.0–3.5 mmol/l. Although $MgSO_4$ is not sedative, it can depress neuromuscular transmission. Reduced patellar reflexes usually precede respiratory depression.

- If respiratory arrest occurs, intubate, ventilate, stop the infusion and give calcium gluconate (10 ml of 10% solution) over 10 min.
- If respiratory depression occurs, give high-flow O_2 (e.g. 6 l/min), stop the infusion and give calcium gluconate (10 ml of 10% solution) over 10 min.

- If the urine output is <100 ml in 4 h, reduce the $MgSO_4$ infusion to 0.5 g/h (2.5 ml/h) and review the fluid balance.
- If reflexes are absent, stop the infusion and restart it once reflexes have returned. Reduce the infusion rate (e.g. to 0.5 g/h = 2.5 ml/h) unless there have been further fits.
- If $MgSO_4$ is <2.0 mmol/l, increase the infusion to 2 g/h for 2 h and recheck.
- If $MgSO_4$ is 3.5–5.0 mmol/l, stop the infusion and restart at 0.5 g/h (2.5 ml/h), providing the urine output is >20 ml/h. If $MgSO_4$ is >5.0 mmol/l, manage as for absent reflexes.
- Continue for at least 24 hours post-fit.

Diazepam (Diazemuls) This is used by some clinicians as an alternative to $MgSO_4$. In the light of the Collaborative Trial (Lancet 1995;345:1455), $MgSO_4$ is likely to be superior.

- Give a bolus: 10 mg IV is given over 2 min, and repeated if convulsions recur.
- Then start an IV infusion: 40 mg in 500 mg normal saline over 24 h titrated according to the level of consciousness. The aim is to overcome restlessness and keep the patient sedated but rousable. Over the next 24 h an infusion of 20 mg diazepam in 500 ml normal saline is given, and slowly reduced.

Side-effects Respiratory depression. If compromised give Flumazanil which comes as 5 ml of 100 µg/ml. The dose is 2 ml (200 µg) over 15 seconds then 1 ml (100 µg) every 60 seconds to a maximum of 1 mg.

Further management

- Involve senior obstetric and anaesthetic staff.
- Monitor the BP.
- Monitor the S_aO_2. Consider measuring ABGs and arranging a CXR if the saturation drops below 93% or there is cough, dyspnoea or tachypnoea.
- Give Ringer's lactate as an IV infusion. The total fluid input (including infusions) should not exceed 80 ml/h. If the urine output drops below 30 ml/h over 4 hours, insert a CVP line. The normal range is 2–8 cmH$_2$O, although the change in the right ventricular pressure to a fluid challenge is probably more important.
- If the CVP is <8 cmH$_2$O, give a 250 ml stat. colloid challenge (e.g. Haemaccel). If there is no increase in urine output and no increase in the CVP, repeat.
- If the CVP is 8–12 cmH$_2$O or there is an increasing trend, give frusemide 20 mg IV stat. Repeat the frusemide in 2 hours if there is no increase in the urine output. If there is still no increase in urine output, set up a dopamine infusion at 3 µg/kg/h. *Do not give NSAIDS.*

- If the CVP is >12 cmH$_2$O, give frusemide 50 mg IV stat. If there is pulmonary oedema, sit the patient up, give high-flow O$_2$ ± vasodilators. Consider transfer to the ITU for a sodium nitroprusside infusion, Swan catheter and IPPV.

(See: ARF, p. 98; ARDS, p. 99, if appropriate.)

HELLP SYNDROME (Br J Obstet Gynaecol 1997:887, Curr Opinion Nephrol 1994:436)

(For differential diagnosis of abnormal LFTs, see p. 125.) ⅓ *amo - DIC*

HELLP is an acronym for haemolysis, elevated liver enzymes (particularly transaminases) and low platelets. It is a variant of pre-eclampsia, affecting 4–12% of those with pre-eclampsia/eclampsia, and is commoner in multigravidae. There may be epigastric pain, nausea, vomiting, and RUQ tenderness. AST rises first (>48 IU/l) then LDH (>164 IU/l). LDH >600 IU/l indicates severe disease. A blood film may show burr cells and polychromasia consistent with haemolysis, although anaemia is uncommon. Platelet transfusion is rarely required with platelets >40×10^9/l, and is likely to be of benefit if <20×10^9/l and delivery is planned. There may be ARF (see p. 98) and DIC (see p. 82), and there is an increased incidence of abruption. There is also an increased incidence (although still rare) of hepatic haematoma and hepatic rupture, leading to profuse intraperitoneal bleeding. Management is to stabilize coagulation, assess fetal well-being and consider the need for delivery. It is generally considered that delivery is appropriate for moderately severe cases, but may be more conservative (with close monitoring) if mild. Postpartum vigilance is required for at least 48 hours. The incidence of recurrence in subsequent pregnancies is about 20%.

DIC - 30%.   *Renal failure 16%.*   *pl-effusion - 6%.*
Abruption - 16%.   *Pulm. edema 6%.   Death - 4%.*

PHAEOCHROMOCYTOMA

This carries a high maternal mortality rate and may mimic pre-eclampsia. Hypertensive crises may be precipitated by anaesthesia or delivery (particularly caesarean section). Diagnosis is by 24 hour urine collection for catecholamines, and tumours should be localized with USS, CT or MRI scanning. Initial treatment is with combined α and β blockers such as phenoxybenzamine 20–40 mg/day PO initially, followed a few days later by propranolol 120–240 mg/day. Hypertensive crises may be treated with sodium nitroprusside. Surgical removal of the tumour can be performed before 24 weeks, but if diagnosed later in pregnancy is best delayed until fetal maturity, when delivery can be performed by elective caesarean section at the same time as tumour removal.

INFECTION

> It is often appropriate to seek bacteriological ± fetal medicine subspecialist advice.

GENERAL

Farm workers

A chlamydia (which causes abortion in sheep), toxoplasma (which cause abortion in cows and sheep) and listeria can all cause abortion in humans. Women who work with farm animals should therefore avoid animal work, particularly in the lambing and calving seasons. This will include vets.

Basic hygiene precautions should be observed by all who are involved at this time. Overalls and boots worn for work should be removed at the house door, and the boots cleaned and left outside. Soiled overalls should be placed directly into the washing machine by the wearer, who should then wash and dry their hands thoroughly. At the end of the season the lambing/calving shed should be thoroughly washed and swept out, and left open to the air for the summer. Handwashing by all who enter the house from the farm at any time is the key to controlling such infection.

Food

- Soft cheeses: only soft cheeses made from pasteurized milk should be eaten, as there is a risk of listeria from unpasteurized milk and its products.
- Raw eggs: these must be avoided, as there is a risk of salmonella (remember puddings). Eggs need to be boiled for 8 minutes to kill salmonella reliably.
- Undercooked or raw meat or pâté may transmit toxoplasma, rarely listeria.
- Unwashed fruit: fruit should always be washed before eating as it may be contaminated with salmonella, toxoplasma or one of several intestinal parasites.

Nurses

Nurses may be concerned about CMV, particularly if they are in contact with small children. Serology is of little benefit, as the presence of antibodies does not necessarily denote immunity (see Table 4.3). Hands should be washed well and often. The risk of CMV is very small.

Travel and vaccinations

Consider aspirin ± graduated compression stockings for long-haul flights. If the woman is visiting a malarial region, give advice on mosquito nets, wearing long sleeves and trousers (tucked into socks), insect-repellent spray, cream, wipes, etc. Antimalarials should be taken (Larium should be avoided if possible, although it may be safe >12 weeks). The risk of vaccinations is likely to be small and probably outweighed by the risk of the disease.

Pets

- There is a risk of toxoplasmosis from *cats*. Women should wear household rubber gloves to clean litter trays and wash their hands afterwards. Better still, they could get someone else to do it! They should also avoid children's sandpits and wear gloves for gardening.
- Adult *dogs* with no diarrhoea do not pose a significant risk.

SPECIFIC INFECTIONS

> **Fetal infection principles**
>
> IgM is not made by the fetus until beyond 20 weeks' gestation. Undetected fetal IgM at birth does not mean that infection has not occurred, and IgG is usually passive unless the baby is older than 1 year. Evidence of infection does not imply damage.

Chickenpox at term   *Refer guideline (RCOG)*

For *chickenpox in early pregnancy*, see Table 4.3.

Severe and even fatal cases of chickenpox can occur in neonates whose mothers develop chickenpox from 7 days before to 1 month after delivery (usually 2 days before to 2 days after). The baby should be given varicella zoster immunoglobulin (VZIG) as soon as possible if maternal symptoms develop. VZIG may be given to babies in contact with chickenpox whose mothers have no history of chickenpox (or no antibodies on testing) and to premature babies (<30 weeks) in contact with chickenpox, irrespective of the mother's history.

Hepatitis

Hepatitis A This has not been associated with significant complications in pregnancy.

Hepatitis B All mothers should be screened antenatally for hepatitis B virus. Transmission is most likely to occur with acute infection (especially in the third trimester), or in the presence of HBeAg. The risk of transmission for HBSAg-positive mothers who are eAg-positive is 90%; for eAg-negative/eAb-negative the risk is 40% and for eAb-positive mothers it is 10%. The baby should be given 0.5 ml hepatitis B immunoglobulin IM into the buttock within 4 hours of birth (or at least within 12 hours) as well as active hepatitis B immunization with 5–10 μg IM to the thigh, repeated at 1 month and at 6 months.

Hepatitis C accounts for 5% of all hepatitides with progression to chronic liver disease in probably all cases after 20–40 years. Progression may be more rapid with other factors (e.g. excess alcohol use). A 6 month course of alpha-interferon and ribovarin may improve the prognosis. Transmission is through contact with unscreened blood or certain blood products, but can be sexual or peri-natal. Vertical transmission is related to viral load but is unlikely in the absence of detected RNA. Primary infection does not increase obstetric complications and pregnancy does not worsen progression. There is no evidence that treatment during pregnancy reduces the chance of transmission and ribovarin is teratogenic. Caesarean section or breast feeding are unlikely to alter the incidence of neo-natal infection. The risks of transmission to medical personnel is low, but the patient should be treated as high risk.

Hepatitis E While uncommon in the UK, hepatitis E infection in pregnancy carries a 30% maternal mortality rate and possible risk of fetal loss.

Herpes simplex virus

An acute attack (primary or secondary) around the time of delivery may lead to a neonatal infection, which may be localized or systemic, occasionally including encephalitis. The risk of infection is greatest with a primary infection, but can occur with recurrence. Antenatal screening at 36 weeks does not predict transmission, and indeed 70% neonatal infections occur to mothers with no overt signs of infection. Membrane rupture in the presence of a primary infection (i.e. within 6 weeks of delivery) is considered by many to be the only indication for caesarean section, providing the operation is carried out within the first 4 hours. It is possible, however, that caesarean section is appropriate in recurrent herpes if active lesions are present (Br J Obstet Gynaecol 1998:255). The very small risk of fetal infection in this situation must be weighed against the risk to the mother of caesarean section. Prescribing continuous oral aciclovir in the last 4 weeks of pregnancy may reduce the number of recurrences, but does not seem to reduce the number of caesarean sections, and is probably not indicated outwith a trial setting (Br J Obstet Gynaecol 1998:275).

Human immunodeficiency virus (HIV)

The HIV retrovirus is transmitted both by contact with body fluids (sexually, needles, unscreened blood transfusions) and by vertical transmission from mother to fetus. After an initial febrile seroconversion illness of varying severity there is a latent phase of up to 8–10 years, with or without the development of progressive generalized lymphadenopathy, and finally symptomatic disease (AIDS). The CD4 count, initially $>500 \times 10^9/l$, falls with disease progression and is usually $<200 \times 10^9/l$ by the time opportunistic infections occur. Such infections include recurrences of vaginal candidiasis and genital herpes. HIV testing should only be carried out after explicit informed consent by the patient following discussion with a named HIV counsellor, who has back-up facilities for the management and support of those found to be infected.

There is some evidence that pregnancy may worsen the course of the disease (Br J Obstet Gynaecol 1998:827) and that HIV infection is associated with a slightly poorer perinatal outcome (Br J Obstet Gynaecol 1998:836). Transmission to the fetus occurs in 13–30% of pregnancies and is greatest in those with late-stage disease as indicated by a low CD4 count or high viral load. It is also higher in those who breast-feed while seroconverting, and those who have traumatic instrumentation in labour. Zidovudine 100 mg PO 5 times a day started between 14 and 34 weeks, continued in labour with a 2 mg/kg loading dose and 1 mg/kg/h IV infusion, and to the neonate 2 mg/kg QID for 6 weeks postdelivery, markedly reduces this vertical transmission. Many centres will use multiple therapies (e.g. AZT and 3TC) to reduce the incidence of viral resistance, although the teratogenic effects are unclear. Protease inhibitors are contraindicated in pregnancy due to teratogenic effects. Caesarean section before labour may also reduce the risk of transmission (or in early labour, providing SRM < 4 hours previously). Breast-feeding should be avoided if safe alternatives are available.

Listeria monocytogenes

This is a rare bacterial infection transmitted by food (usually soft ripe cheeses, pâté, cooked–chilled meals and ready-to-eat foods which have not been thoroughly cooked). Following an initial gastroenteritis, which may be fleeting, bacteraemia results in bacilli crossing the placenta, leading to amnionitis, preterm labour (which may result in still birth) or spontaneous abortion. There may be meconium, neonatal jaundice, conjunctivitis or meningoencephalitis. Diagnosis is made by blood culture or by culture of liquor or placenta. Treatment is with high-dose amoxycillin or erythromycin.

Group B β-haemolytic streptococci

Between 5% and 20% of women carry this organism, which is a bowel commensal, in the vagina. It is associated with preterm prelabour and preterm rupture of the membranes. About 50% of babies become colonized at delivery, but only about 1% of these develop infection. The mortality from infection may be up to 80%, with 50% of those surviving meningitis having subsequent neurological impairment. Antenatal screening is not indicated in the UK (initial screen positives may become negative, and vice versa), but those with known infection should receive intrapartum antibiotics (e.g. amoxycillin or erythromycin). There is no evidence to support antenatal treatment of asymptomatic carriers, as carriage is rapidly re-established following treatment.

TABLE 4.3 Infections in pregnancy

Agent	Epidemiology	Maternal features	Fetal features	Risk	Investigation	Treatment	Recurrence
Rubella (RNA virus)	Person to person. Infectious from 7 days before to 4 days after onset of rash. Incubation 14–21 days. UK immunity now 97% and congenital infection is rare	Mild maculopapular rash. May be asymptomatic in adults, but may include thrombocytopenia and arthralgia	IUGR, ↓platelets, hepatosplenomegaly, jaundice, deafness, CHD (VSD, PDA), mental retardation, cataracts, microphthalmia, abortion, microcephaly and cerebral palsy	Risk of affected fetus: <4 weeks, 50% 5–8 weeks, 25% 9–12 weeks, 10% >13 weeks, 1% Early in utero diagnosis is unreliable, but IgM in fetal blood >22 weeks is likely to be significant	A fourfold ↑IgG 28 days postexposure (raised level <1 days = previous exposure). Take 1st specimen <10 days before rash and 2nd specimen 14–21 days later	Consider TOP if <12 weeks PN vaccination if not immune (i.e. antibodies <15 IU (avoid pregnancy for 1 month)	Probably minimal significance
Toxoplasmosis (protozoan, Toxoplasma gondii)	From cats, uncooked meats and unwashed fruits Incubation <2 days Seroprevalence 20–70%	May have fever, rash and lymphadenopathy. But ≈80% are asymptomatic	Hydrocephalus, chorioretinitis, intracranial calcification, ↓platelets	<12 weeks transmission is 10–25%, of which 75% will be severely affected 12–28 weeks transmission is 54%, of which 25% will be severely affected >28 weeks transmission is 65–90%, of which ≪10% will be severely affected	↑ Maternal IgM fourfold over 4 weeks (may be +ve for up to 1 year). Even if amniotic fluid positive, 90% are normal. FBS also unreliable test	Consider TOP only if primary infection <20 weeks There is evidence that giving Spiramycin and Pyrimethamine may be of benefit (Lancet 1994; 344:36)	Probably no significant risk
CMV (herpes virus)	Person to person Low infectivity Incubation 21 days Seroprevalence 50%.	Nearly always asymptomatic	Hepatosplenomegaly, ↓platelets, IUGR, microcephaly, sensorineural deafness, CP, chorioretinitis, hydrops fetalis, exomphalos	40% fetuses infected. Risk unaffected by gestation Of these, 90% are normal at birth, although 20% develop late sequelae Of the 10% who are symptomatic, 33% die and the rest have long-term problems	↑ Maternal IgM and IgG, or culture/PCR of maternal urine In utero diagnosis of infection may be possible by amniotic fluid culture an PCR 4–6 weeks after infection, but false-negative rate is 45%. As before, being infected does not	Even primary infection proven by amnio-culture carries only a 10–25% risk of severe abnormality; therefore counselling regarding TOP is difficult (i.e. as 75–90% are normal) Prevent in those at risk (frequent contact with	Reactivation is common and accounts for more neonatal problems in total than primary infection Risk of fetal infection with reactivation is <1%

TABLE 4.3 Infections in pregnancy (cont'd)

Agent	Epidemiology	Maternal features	Fetal features	Risk	Investigation	Treatment	Recurrence
Parvovirus B₁₉	Respiratory transmission, especially in those dealing with children. Highly infectious. Incubation 4–20 days Seroprevalence 50%	Erythema infectiosum (slapped cheek disease) May be asymptomatic	Aplastic anaemia, hydrops fetalis and myocarditis ± fetal loss (if <20 weeks) Transmission <20 weeks = 10% of which are lost If >20 weeks, transmission 60%, but no adverse affects have been demonstrated	If less than 20 weeks and fetus survives the infection (≈ 90%) it is likely to result in a healthy live birth (i.e. no association with structural abnormalities even after 7–10 year follow up Br J Obstet Gynaecol 1998:174) Hydrops may present on USS after 3–9 weeks, following initial infection	↑IgM with clinical illness (for 3 months) and ↑IgG after 7 days B₁₉ virus can be demonstrated by PCR following FBS	Intrauterine transfusion may be possible, and hydropic fetuses should be referred to a fetal medicine unit	Unknown
Chickenpox (varicella zoster virus)	Person to person Highly infectious Incubation 10–20 days Seroprevalence >90%	Papules and pustules Increased severity in pregnancy, including increased risk of varicella pneumonia. Consider treating mother with Acyclovir if unwell, although fetal effects unknown	Limb hypoplasia, skin scarring, IUGR, neurological abnormalities and hydrops fetalis	25% transmission Probably <1–2% have problems if <20 weeks No structural problems >20 weeks See Chickenpox at Term, p. 135	FBS for IgM has low sensitivity	Give zoster immunoglobulin if <10 days from contact or <4 days from onset of rash, although the benefits are not proven	Shingles in mother carries no risk, but a non-immune mother coming into contact with shingles does carry a risk

mean fetus is affected
Neonatal diagnosis from urine at <3 weeks

children or known infection) by washing hands, particularly after saliva contact

PSYCHIATRIC PROBLEMS IN THE PUERPERIUM

The postnatal blues

This occurs in >50% of women, usually beginning on days 2–4, peaking at days 4–6 and lasting for 2–7 days. This is a mood disturbance rather than a mood illness, which may have a hormonal basis and is unrelated to obstetric or cultural factors. There is emotional lability, tearfulness, sadness, sleep disturbance, poor concentration, restlessness and headaches. The mother may feel vulnerable and/or rejected, and may show undue concern for the baby. Treatment is with reassurance. Antenatal preparation may be of help.

Postnatal depression

The incidence is 25% of women in the first postnatal year, with the peak onset around weeks 3–4. In two-thirds, the illness is self-limiting; in one-third it may be sustained or severe. There are the usual features of depression, but particularly increased irritability, tiredness, decreased libido, guilt at not loving or caring enough for the baby, inability to cope with the baby or undue anxieties over the baby's health and feeding. It is more likely in those who have had adverse life events shortly before or during pregnancy, those in marital conflict and those ambivalent to motherhood. It is not related to obstetric factors, but may be associated with a past history of depression. Treatment depends on severity, circumstances and patient preferences, but includes brief psychotherapy, supportive psychotherapy, counselling and antidepressants. The outcome is generally good.

Puerperal psychosis

There is an incidence of 1:500 to 1:800 deliveries, beginning around days 3–7 and peaking at 2 weeks. There may be serious risks to both the mother and child. One study has suggested that 5% of patients commit suicide and 4% kill their baby. There are variable psychotic symptoms, sometimes superimposed upon postnatal blues. The clinical picture is a shifting one, often ushered in by one or two nights' insomnia. Mood abnormality is common and the mother may be suspicious, sometimes denying the pregnancy and baby. There may be delusions, hallucinations, confusion and cognitive impairment. It is associated with a past history of psychosis (especially manic depression), with being unmarried, having a caesarean section, developing an infection or suffering a perinatal death. Mother and baby should be admitted to hospital, ideally to a mother and baby unit. The prognosis is good for the incident episode, particularly if the family is supportive. Of those who become pregnant again, 20% will develop another puerperal psychosis. Overall, 50% will have another psychotic episode at some time in their life.

RENAL DISORDERS

> In pregnancy, there is an increase in the size of both kidneys and dilatation of the ureter and renal pelvis. This is greater on the right than the left because of the dextro-rotation of the uterus. There is also an increase in creatinine clearance due to the increased GFR (maximum in the second trimester). Urea should be <4.5 mmol/l and creatinine <75 μmol/l (see also ARF, p. 98).

Infection

UTIs occur in 3–7% of pregnancies and, if untreated, may lead to septicaemia and premature labour. Asymptomatic bacteriuria should be treated in all pregnant women as there is a 30–40% risk of developing a symptomatic UTI. Treat pyelonephritis aggressively, including using aminoglycosides for severe Gram-negative infection (e.g. gentamicin, see p. 104).

Obstruction

Acute hydronephrosis is characterized by loin pain, ureteric colic, sterile urine and a renal USS showing dilatation of the renal tract greater than in normal pregnancy. If the symptoms are not settling and the USS does not demonstrate the cause of the obstruction consider a limited IVU. Treatment is with ureteric stenting or nephrostomy. There may be no obvious cause of obstruction and complete resolution may occur following delivery. Renal tract calculi are associated with an increased incidence of UTIs but otherwise do not usually affect pregnancy (unless obstruction is severe).

Previous surgery

This does not usually affect pregnancy. Congenital malformations of the urinary tract may be associated with genital tract malformations. A pelvic kidney may rarely cause obstruction at delivery.

Chronic renal disease in pregnancy

The prognosis is best if renal function and BP are normal. If the plasma creatinine is <125 μmol/l the maternal and perinatal outcome is usually good. If plasma creatinine is >250 μmol/l there is usually amenorrhoea and, if pregnancy occurs, there may be a risk of renal deterioration (therefore consider TOP). Between these levels women should be advised that pregnancy may cause their renal function to deteriorate and that there are also risks to the fetus (mainly IUGR). Pre-existing hypertension, proteinuria and a pre-pregnancy GFR <70 ml/min are also associated with a poorer maternal and fetal outcome. Some renal diseases carry a worse prognosis than others (seek specialist advice).

Pre-pregnancy counselling is ideal. The patient should be seen frequently antenatally, particularly in the third trimester. Check BP (treat aggressively), U&E, plasma protein, urinalysis and MSUs at each visit and send 24 hour urine collections each month for protein and creatinine clearance. Close fetal monitoring is important in the third trimester. The patient should be admitted if there is deteriorating creatinine clearance, increasing proteinuria, hypertension >140/90 mmHg, evidence of fetal compromise or rapidly increasing or decreasing maternal weight.

Serial changes in creatinine clearance are more important than a single low value. It is difficult to distinguish pre-eclampsia from increasing renal compromise as both may present with hypertension and proteinuria. As pre-eclampsia is also associated with a long-term deterioration in renal function, the treatment is similar and involves treatment of the hypertension (see p. 127), assessment of the fetus and delivery if possible. If the pregnancy progresses uneventfully to 38 weeks it may be advisable to consider induction.

Pregnancy should be discouraged in patients on dialysis (despite most patients being amenorrhoeic, the need for contraception should be emphasized). If pregnancy does occur, consider TOP. If pregnancy continues, electrolytes should be stabilized within the normal pregnant range, although the prognosis for the fetus is poor (miscarriage in the second trimester is common).

Pregnancy in patients with renal transplant

Women should be advised to wait for 1 year following transplant before conceiving. If well, with no evidence of hypertension, proteinuria or transplant rejection, there is unlikely to be any increased risk of transplant failure. There should be regular assessment, with FBC, U&E, creatinine clearance, calcium, phosphate and plasma proteins. Vitamin D, calcium, iron and folate supplements are recommended. CMV, HBV and Hep C titres should be checked. Monitor for bacteriuria. Proteinuria may occur around term but, in the absence of hypertension, is not significant. Pre-eclampsia is particularly difficult to diagnose, as proteinuria and urate levels do not behave as expected. Immunosuppressant therapy should be kept to the lowest dose possible as all these drugs may be teratogenic in high doses. Signs of transplant rejection are fever, oliguria and deteriorating renal function.

Aim for a vaginal delivery, with careful attention to fluid balance in labour. Give antibiotics to cover all surgical procedures (including episiotomy repair). Steroid cover is required as patients are invariably taking prednisolone. The ectopic kidney does not usually obstruct labour. Care should be taken to avoid damage to the kidney or ureter if caesarean section is carried out, and a classical caesarean section may be required.

The fetus is at risk of IUGR, congenital infection, adrenal insufficiency, thymic atrophy, septicaemia and bone marrow hypoplasia. There is no increased risk of congenital anomalies in women on the conventional levels of immunosuppressants, although the data are limited. It is not yet clear if there are long-term effects on the offspring.

RESPIRATORY DISORDERS

Breathlessness

Breathlessness due to the physiological increase in ventilation is a common symptom in pregnancy. This is due partly to the effect of progesterone and partly to a raised diaphragm, which occurs even before the uterus causes direct physical pressure. A normal CXR and physical examination virtually excludes a pathological problem in the absence of other symptoms.

Asthma

Asthma affects 3% of women in pregnancy. In most the disease is unchanged, but it may improve or, less commonly, deteriorate. Treatment is similar to that in the non-pregnant patient and patients already established on treatment should continue. Peak flow rates should be monitored. Inhaled β-sympathomimetics and inhaled steroids are safe. Oral steroids and theophylline are safe, but theophylline is cleared rapidly due to the increased GFR.

Mild asthma should be treated with inhaled β-sympathomimetics (e.g. salbutamol, two puffs as required). If this is required more than once per day, then give prophylaxis with inhaled steroids (e.g. Becotide, two puffs QID). If this is ineffective, then a short course of oral prednisolone 40 mg/day may be necessary. Chest infections should be treated with antibiotics as required.

Asthma is rarely a problem in labour. Those who have been on continuous oral steroid therapy for more than 3 weeks in the previous year should receive intrapartum prophylaxis with hydrocortisone 100 mg QID IV. PGF-2α and ergometrine should be avoided. NSAIDs should be used with caution.

Management of severe acute asthma

A peak flow of <200 l/min indicates severe obstruction. The ABGs initially show a respiratory alkalosis with a normal O_2, decreased CO_2 and increased pH, but later progress to respiratory acidosis with increased CO_2, decreased O_2 and decreased pH.

- Give nebulized salbutamol 5 mg in 5 ml with O_2 at 10 l/min. If there is no response, give nebulized ipratropium bromide 0.5 mg in 2 ml.
- Establish IV access and give hydrocortisone 200 mg IV 6 hourly.
- If severe, consider aminophylline only if not already taking oral theophyllines. Give aminophylline 250 mg (i.e. 10 ml) slowly IV (over 10 min) with ECG monitoring, followed by an IV infusion at 500 µg/kg/h — add 250 mg to 500 ml normal saline. Take the patient's weight (in kg) and run the IV infusion at this in ml/h (e.g. if the patient weighs 65 kg then run the infusion at 65 ml/h).
- Intubate if there is maternal exhaustion, systolic BP <90 mmHg or deteriorating ABGs (P_aO_2 < 6.5 kPa, P_aCO_2 > 6.5 kPa or pH < 7.3).
- Use IPPV with humidified oxygen through a large-bore endotracheal tube ± sedation to minimize barotrauma.
- Give antibiotics and physiotherapy in the longer term if there is infection.

Cystic fibrosis

Increasingly, women with cystic fibrosis are reaching childbearing age. The partner should be screened for the known mutant alleles and, if positive, amniocentesis offered (see p. 28). Maternal mortality is no different from the mortality amongst non-pregnant cystic fibrosis sufferers. Perinatal mortality, however, is increased. Pregnancy is most likely to be successful if the woman's nutritional status is good and she does not have emphysema or cor pulmonale. The pregnancy should be monitored carefully, and diabetes mellitus or liver disease treated if present. There is increased sodium loss in sweat, and this may lead to hypovolaemia in labour (although if there is cor pulmonale then care should be taken to avoid overhydration). There is a small risk of intrapartum pneumothorax. Regional anaesthesia is preferred to GA if pulmonary function is satisfactory.

Sarcoidosis

The course of sarcoidosis is not altered by pregnancy. There is a slight risk of exacerbation in the puerperium, but unless the disease is severe there is no contraindication to pregnancy. There is no special treatment required and no risk of transmission to the fetus.

Pneumothorax and pneumomediastinum

These occur more frequently in labour than at other times in individuals with an increased susceptibility. Pneumomediastinum may occur in association with vomiting, leading to subcutaneous emphysema over the thorax. A CXR shows absent lung markings and a mediastinal shift in the pneumothorax, and air in the subcutaneous tissues in the pneumomediastinum. If more than 30% of the lung is collapsed then a chest drain is required. Pneumomediastinum will improve spontaneously. If there has been a pneumothorax during pregnancy then elective forceps delivery should be carried out to minimise the risk of recurrence.

THROMBOCYTOPENIA

> In normal pregnancies there is a gradual decrease in the platelet count, although the majority will still lie within the normal range. A high platelet count postnatally is usually physiological, but recheck.

MATERNAL THROMBOCYTOPENIA IN PREGNANCY

Pregnancy associated thrombocytopenia

In the second half of 8% of normal pregnancies there is a mild thrombocytopenia (platelet count $100–150 \times 10^9$/l) which is not associated with any risk to the mother or fetus.

Pre-eclampsia and HELLP syndrome

See pages 130 and 133.

Disseminated intravascular coagulation (DIC)

See page 82.

Autoimmune thrombocytopenic purpura

This is the commonest cause of thrombocytopenia in early pregnancy (but can also arise in later pregnancy) and may be acute or chronic. There is an isolated thrombocytopenia without other haematological upset, splenomegaly or lymphadenopathy. Antiplatelet antibodies may be detected, but their absence does not exclude AITP. These antibodies may cross the placenta and cause fetal thrombocytopenia, although this is rarely associated with long-term morbidity (unlike alloimmune thrombocytopenia – see below). No treatment is required in the absence of bleeding, providing the platelet count remains above $50 \times 10^9/l$. If the platelet count falls below this level, give steroids (e.g. prednisolone 40 mg/ day), although the response is usually poor. An alternative is an immunoglobulin IV infusion (1 g/kg over 8 hours) with a response usually seen within 48 hours. Avoid splenectomy in pregnancy. If there is mucous membrane bleeding, or if delivery is likely to occur before there is a response to these treatments, then platelet transfusions are required. Platelets should be available in women with severe thrombocytopenia at delivery; there is little risk of bleeding from the placental site, but bleeding from incisions and lacerations may be marked.

Severe fetal thrombocytopenia secondary to antibody transfer across the placenta may be associated with intracranial haemorrhage during delivery. It is, however, very difficult to predict the fetal platelet count from the maternal platelet count. The fetal platelet count can be assessed by cordocentesis at 38 weeks in women with a platelet count $<100 \times 10^9/l$, but this carries potential fetal risks. As the overall perinatal mortality rate in AITP patients is similar to that in the normal population, it would seem reasonable to allow vaginal delivery in most women. Traumatic delivery, FBS and fetal scalp electrode should be avoided. Cord blood should be taken at delivery to measure the neonatal platelet count. This should also be done in women who have had a splenectomy for AITP, who may still have circulating antiplatelet antibodies.

Other conditions

Thrombocytopenia may also occur with infection, drugs, alcohol, malignant infiltration of bone marrow, or be associated with megaloblastic anaemia, SLE (see p. 111) or HIV infection (see p. 136).

ALLOIMMUNE THROMBOCYTOPENIA

This is a rare disorder in which there are maternal antibodies to fetal platelets (similar to Rhesus disease). The maternal platelet level is normal, but there may be profound fetal thrombocytopenia and antenatal or intrapartum intracranial bleeds. The diagnosis should be suspected when a previous child has had neonatal thrombocytopenia (usually associated with cerebral damage) and maternal antiplatelet antibodies have been identified (usually to the HPA-1a antigen). Treatment is controversial, but fetal platelet measurement by cordocentesis at 22 weeks has been used to assess the need for weekly maternal IV IgG (1 g/kg). This carries risks however and, although expensive, it is probably most appropriate to give maternal IV IgG regularly without performing any invasive fetal procedure. Maternal steroid administration is unlikely to increase platelet levels. Antenatal monitoring with USS is important, looking particularly for intracranial bleeding, and delivery should probably be by caesarean section for all. There is a 75–95% recurrence in subsequent pregnancies.

THROMBOEMBOLIC DISEASE

> Normal pregnancy contributes to all three components of Virchow's triad. Venous thromboembolism is the commonest direct cause of maternal mortality in the UK (Confidential Enquiry into Maternal Deaths in the UK 1994–1996). The incidence of PTE is 0.3–1.2% of all pregnancies, with just over 40% of cases occurring antenatally, often in the first trimester. Over 80% of DVTs in pregnancy are left sided and >70% are ileofemoral (unlike in non-pregnant patients). Risk factors include obesity, age >35 years, high parity, previous thromboembolism, immobility, pre-eclampsia, varicose veins, congenital or acquired thrombophilia, intercurrent infection and caesarean section (particularly emergency caesarean section).

Diagnosis of DVT
DVT may be asymptomatic; in addition to the traditional symptoms and signs, it may also present with lower abdominal pain. It is essential to make a definitive diagnosis if possible. Duplex Doppler ultrasound is particularly useful for identifying femoral vein thromboses, although iliac veins are less easily seen. This is safe and should be the first-line investigation. Venography is better, but has the disadvantage of radiation exposure and should be carried out if the Doppler scan gives equivocal results or is not available. Breast-feeding following contrast injection is safe.

Diagnosis of pulmonary embolism
(If collapsed, see Cardiorespiratory Arrest, p. 102.)
  Pleuritic chest pain, breathlessness, cough and haemoptysis are the major symptoms. These may be mild or associated with collapse and cardiopulmonary arrest. The ECG is frequently normal and the CXR is usually normal but may

show a raised hemidiaphragm, atelectasis, reduced vascular markings, effusions or infiltrates. ABGs may show hyperventilation ($PCO_2 < 4.5$ kPa) and decreased O_2 exchange (e.g. $PO2 < 8$ kPa). A VQ scan is required. Pregnancy is not a contraindication to this investigation and the risks are far outweighed by the benefits of diagnosis. A normal scan virtually excludes the diagnosis of pulmonary embolism. If equivocal, arrange duplex Doppler ultrasound of legs.

Management of DVT or pulmonary embolism
Start treatment as soon as clinical suspicion arises; do not wait for a definitive diagnosis. Check a baseline coagulation screen and platelets. Instead of traditional heparin 5000 IU IV stat followed by a 1000 IU/h IV infusion with checking of the APTT after 6 hours and adjusting the infusion rate to keep the APTT 1.5–2 times the control, it may be reasonable to use low-molecular-weight heparin (e.g. enoxaparin 1 mg/kg BD). Continue this in labour and the puerperium. Postnatally the patient may wish to continue with SC heparin or start warfarin 10 mg PO on days 3 and 4, adjusting the dose thereafter to keep the INR at 2–2.5 and stopping the heparin once the INR is stable. Warfarin does not cross into breast milk in significant quantities. Anticoagulation should be continued until at least 6, and ideally 12, weeks postpartum and for at least 12 weeks if the event occurred postnatally. Treatment with streptokinase or caval filters may be useful in certain circumstances. Once anticoagulants are stopped, women should be screened for thrombophilia.

Management of those with a previous thromboembolic history
Women who have had a single episode of DVT/PTE should be screened for thrombophilia. This can only be carried out comprehensively distant from the clotting event and after stopping anticoagulant medication. Check for the congenital thrombophilias – activated protein C resistance (if present, test for the factor V Leiden mutation), antithrombin, protein C and protein S deficiency – as well as the antiphospholipid syndrome (see p. 111), which may be associated with an increased risk of fetal loss (those homozygous for the factor V Leiden mutation may also have a less optimum fetal outcome). More recently the prothrombin gene variant and hyperhomocystinaemia have also been associated with an increased risk of venous thromboembolic disease. If the screen is negative, and the event occurred outside pregnancy, and was not severe, thromboprophylaxis may not be required. If the event occurred during pregnancy and the thrombophilia screen is negative then prophylaxis during pregnancy may be considered as below, and should probably be given postpartum.

Those who have had multiple thromboembolic events should commence antenatal prophylaxis, as below, 4–6 weeks in advance of the gestation at which their previous episode occurred, or sooner if additional risk factors, and continue postpartum. Those with congenital thrombophilia and previous venous thromboembolic event should have prophylaxis antenatally, particularly those with antithrombin III deficiency, and they should certainly have postnatal prophylaxis. This also applies to women with a single episode of DVT/PTE together with a positive family history, even if the thrombophilia screen is negative. Patients with lupus anticoagulant or anticardiolipin antibodies should probably receive postpartum prophylaxis, and if they have a previous history of DVT/PTE, they should probably receive antenatal prophylaxis as well. Better data on this controversial area are expected after completion of the Assessment of the Prevention of Pulmonary Embolism and deep venous thrombosis with Low molecular weight hEparin (APPLE) trial.

Antenatal prophylaxis Use unfractionated heparin 7500–10 000 IU SC BD or low-molecular-weight (LMW) heparin (enoxaparin 40 mg, dalteparin 5000 IU) SC once daily. LMW heparin can be monitored by checking anti-factor Xa activity, which should be 0.2–0.4 IU/ml for prophylaxis, but this is only really necessary with antithrombin deficiency where therapeutic doses of anticoagulant are used. Platelet counts should be checked regularly because of the risk of heparin-induced thrombocytopenia.

Postnatal prophylaxis Use unfractionated heparin 7500 IU SC BD or LMW heparin (enoxaparin 40 mg, dalteparin 5000 IU) SC once daily. Consider changing to warfarin 2–3 days after delivery (heparin should be continued until the INR is 2–2.5). Treat for 6–12 weeks.

Risks of antenatal prophylaxis

Patients already on warfarin before pregnancy should be reviewed and should be changed to SC heparin. Although it has been traditional to maintain patients with mechanical prosthetic heart valves on warfarin because of the adverse fetal effects (see below) there is now a view that therapeutic heparin may be the better treatment (Br J Obstet Gynaecol 1998:683). This should be changed to IV heparin at 37 weeks. Some clinicians would consider full-dose SC heparin for this group over the period of organogenesis (5–12 weeks).

Those who have a significant risk of thromboembolism should not be denied prophylaxis. Heparin may be associated with maternal thrombocytopenia and platelet counts should be monitored regularly during treatment. Long-term heparin therapy is also associated with maternal osteoporosis (fracture risk 1–2%), and women should be made aware of this risk. This is less with LMW heparin. Heparin does not cross the placenta. The specific teratogenic risk of warfarin treatment in the first trimester is uncertain. Although the miscarriage rate is relatively high (≈30%), the incidence of skeletal, optic and mental retardation is probably lower than was previously thought. There is also a risk of fetal intracerebral haemorrhage in later pregnancy. Warfarin is safe during breast-feeding.

> **Remember**
>
> Warfarin may be reversed in the acute situation with 2–4 U of FFP IV stat.
> Heparin may be reversed with protamine sulphate 1 mg/100 U to a maximum of
> 50 mg (10–15 mg usually suffices).

Postnatal risk assessment

 **If you have performed a caesarean section or instrumental
delivery, it is your duty to prescribe thromboprophylaxis.**

The risks of thromboembolism should be assessed in all patients following
caesarean section. Those at low risk should be mobilized early and receive
appropriate hydration. Those at moderate risk (i.e. one or more risk factor,
see below) should receive unfractionated heparin 5000 IU SC BD for 5 days
or until mobile.

It is also essential to consider prophylaxis in those who have had vaginal
deliveries, whether instrumental or not.

Low risk: early mobilization and hydration

- Elective caesarean section; uncomplicated pregnancy and no other risk factors

Moderate risk: heparin (e.g. heparin 5000 U BD or enoxaparin 20 mg)
and TED graduated compression stockings

- Age >35 years
- Obesity (>80 kg)
- Para 4 or more
- Gross varicose veins
- Current infection
- Pre-eclampsia
- Immobility prior to surgery (>4 days)
- Major current illness (e.g. heart or lung disease, cancer, inflammatory bowel
  disease, nephrotic syndrome)
- Emergency caesarean section in labour

High risk: heparin (e.g. heparin 5000 U TID or enoxaparin 40 mg)
and TED graduated compression stockings

- A patient with three or more moderate risk factors (above)
- Extended major pelvic or abdominal surgery (e.g. caesarean, hysterectomy)
- Patients with a personal or family history of deep vein thrombosis, pulmonary
  embolism or thrombophilia, paralysis of lower limbs
- Patients with antiphospholipid antibody (cardiolipin antibody or lupus
  anticoagulant)

THYROID DISORDERS

> In the western world 1% of pregnant women are affected by thyroid disease, with hypothyroidism being commoner than hyperthyroidism. The fetal thyroid gland is active and secretes thyroid hormones from the 12th week. It is independent of maternal control, although maternal thyroid hormones do cross the placenta.

Measure:

- Free T4 (normal range: 11–23 pmol/l in the first and second trimesters, 7–15 pmol/l in the third trimester),
- Free T3 (normal range 4–8.5 pmol/l in first and second trimesters, 3–5 pmol/l in the third trimester)
- TSH (normal range 0.3–5.0 mU/l).

Hypothyroidism

This may present with fatigue, hair loss, dry skin, abnormal weight gain, poor appetite, cold intolerance, bradycardia and delayed tendon reflexes. If untreated there is double the rate of spontaneous abortions and SBs compared to the normal population, as well as a risk of fetal neurological impairment. There is minimal fetal risk if the mother is euthyroid. Commence thyroxine 0.2 mg/day PO. Monitor thyroid function monthly, aiming to keep TSH within the normal range and free T4 at the upper end of the normal range. If already on treatment and euthyroid at booking, the dose need not be increased.

Fetal hypothyroidism This may occur when the mother carries antithyroid antibodies or is receiving antithyroid drugs.

Thyrotoxicosis

This presents with weight loss, exophthalmos, tachycardia and restlessness. It is usually due to Graves' disease, but may occur secondary to toxic thyroid adenoma or multinodular goitre. Untreated thyrotoxicosis is associated with 48% fetal mortality and a risk of maternal thyroid crisis at delivery. Well-controlled hyperthyroidism is not associated with an increase in fetal anomalies, but there is a tendency for babies to be small for gestational age. Graves' disease usually improves during pregnancy.

Management

- hCG has some thyroid stimulating activity and pregnancy (particularly molar pregnancy) may result in biochemical hyperthyroidism with normal or low TSH levels. If there are no clinical features of thyrotoxicosis in this instance, however, then probably no treatment is required.

- Fetal thyrotoxicosis may occur in 10% of women with current or treated Graves' disease, although oral antithyroid treatment does reduce fetal T4 production. Carry out serial USS for growth, goitre and fetal heart rate. Neonates should be examined for goitre and cord T4 and TSH checked.
- Check antithyroid antibodies (thyroid stimulating antibody is present in Graves' disease). Commence carbimazole 15 mg PO TID or propylthiouracil 150 mg PO TID for 4–5 weeks, and then gradually reduce to the lowest possible dose in order to maintain euthyroid level, preferably with carbimazole <10 mg/day or propylthiouracil <150 mg/day. In the acute phase, if there is a significant tachycardia, β blockers may be added. Thyroid function should be checked at least monthly, aiming to keep TSH within the normal range and free T4 at the upper end of the normal range. Radioactive iodine is absolutely contraindicated, and surgery is indicated only for those with very large goitre, those with poor oral compliance and when malignancy is suspected. Carbimazole and propylthiouracil cross the placenta and can potentially cause fetal thyroid suppression. In low doses, however, this is rarely significant.

Thyroid crisis

This is rare, but may occur in association with stress (e.g. labour) and presents with fever, tachycardia, atrial fibrillation, psychosis and coma. It carries a 10% mortality. Treat with propylthiouracil 1000 mg PO stat. initially followed by 200 mg QID (which can be given by nasogastric tube if necessary). One hour after the first dose, give potassium iodide 500 mg IV infusion TID (or orally QID). If there is no evidence of heart failure, give propranolol 0.5 mg IV stat. followed by 0.5 mg/min IV infusion or 80 mg TID PO. Chlorpromazine 25–50 mg 8-hourly PO or IV will treat psychosis and have a hypothermic effect. Rehydrate with IV fluids (e.g. dextrose) and treat heart failure with digoxin and diuretics.

Postpartum thyroiditis

This occurs following 5–10% of all pregnancies, with initial hyperthyroidism (low technetium uptake, unlike in Graves' disease) followed by hypothyroidism (around 1–3 months, therefore do not confuse with depression) and then recovery. Symptoms of hyperthyroidism may be treated with propranolol (antithyroid drugs accelerate the appearance of hypothyroidism). Treat hypothyroidism with thyroxine as above, withdrawing around 6 months postnatally. A small proportion may require long-term treatment or may develop hypothyroidism later in life.

GYNAECOLOGY

ABORTION

INDUCED ABORTION (TERMINATION OF PREGNANCY)

> Strictly speaking this refers to any pregnancy induced at <24 weeks (UK) or <500 g (WHO). Viability has been achieved lower than these parameters so that in reality the definitions are blurred.

Abortion is legal in the UK under the Abortion Act (1967):

Class A   to save the mother's life,

Class B   to prevent grave permanent injury to the mother's physical or mental health,

Class C   if <24 weeks, to avoid injury to the physical or mental health of the mother,

Class D   if <24 weeks, to avoid injury to the physical or mental health of the existing child(ren),

Class E   if the child is likely to be severely physically or mentally handicapped.

Counselling for 'social' (class C) terminations

Tell me all about it. Does he know and what does he think? How do you get on together? Does anyone else know and what did they say? What do you think? How would you manage if you went ahead with the pregnancy? And how would you feel after the abortion? Would you ever consider having children in the future? Have you considered adoption? What about contraception afterwards? What about follow-up for counselling again?

The woman must be aware that there is a possibility, albeit rare, that infection after TOP may lead to tubal occlusion and secondary infertility. There is also a failure rate and either a clinical follow-up or pregnancy test 2–6 weeks after the termination is important. (*Note*: A pregnancy test may be positive for up to 4 weeks despite successful TOP.) It is important to either screen for and treat infections (including chlamydia), or treat all prophylactically (e.g. Metronidazole 1 g PR (or 800 mg PO) and Azithromycin 1 g PO).

Method

It is important to confirm that the woman is pregnant and to establish the gestation either clinically or by USS. Blood should be sent for grouping and antibodies, and anti-D given after termination to Rhesus-negative women. Options (if available) should be explained and the woman given the choice as outlined below:

- <9 weeks: suction evacuation or medical termination.
- 9–12 weeks: suction termination only.
- >12 weeks: medical termination only.

(*Note*: Some experienced practitioners will consider surgical dilatation and evacuation up to 18 weeks' gestation.)

Suction termination

Surgery is usually carried out under GA (LA is occasionally an option) using cervical dilators and rigid or flexible suction curettes (see p. 220). Definite products of conception must be seen at operation. A 1 mg Cervagem pessary PV (or misoprostol 400–800 µg PV; Br J Obstet Gynaecol 1998:413) should be given to all women 2–4 hours prior to their operation. [*Note*: Misoprostol is effective, but currently is unlicensed.]

Medical termination (RCOG Guideline No. 11, 1997)

First trimester Mifepristone 200–600 mg PO is given on day 1. The patient is admitted to hospital 36–48 hours later and given a 0.5–1 mg Cervagem pessary (or misoprostol 800 µg PV). Overall, 80% will pass products of conception in the following 4 hours; this should be confirmed by clinical inspection and speculum examination before discharge; 94% will abort spontaneously (Br Med J 1993:532); and most will bleed for a total of 10 days. Follow-up should be arranged for 2 weeks to ensure that bleeding has settled and to confirm complete abortion by bimanual examination. If in doubt, USS is useful. Retained products can almost always be managed conservatively, unless bleeding is particularly heavy. Less than 5% of patients require ERPOC.

Second trimester Mifepristone 200–600 mg PO is given on day 1, and the patient admitted to hospital 36–48 hours later and given a 1 mg Cervagem pessary (misoprostol 800 µg PV is an alternative). She is then fasted until abortion occurs and an IV infusion is set up if more than 6 hours pass. Further Cervagem pessaries are inserted 6 hourly (or misoprostol 400 µg PO 3 hourly to a maximum of 4 oral doses if being used as the alternative) until the fetus is expelled or until 24 hours have passed (96% will abort by 24 hours, mean 8 hours). If still not aborted, give pessaries 3 hourly for the next 12 hours (Br J Obstet Gynaecol 193:758). It is important to ensure that the placenta is complete and that the uterus is well contracted on bimanual examination. If the placenta is retained, wait at least 1 hour, unless bleeding is heavy. Approximately 6% will require an ERPOC. Follow-up is as above.

SPONTANEOUS ABORTION (MISCARRIAGE)

- Spontaneous abortion is the loss of a pregnancy before 24 weeks' gestation. It is most common in the first trimester and is said to occur in ≈25% of all pregnancies.
- The word 'abortion' has connotations of induced abortion and should not be used for miscarriage. The term 'blighted ovum' is dreadful and should be discarded.
- Extreme care must be taken not to advise uterine evacuation if there is any possibility of viability.
- Do not assume that the pregnancy is non-viable simply because the gestation does not agree with the expected dates.
- There should also be a low threshold of suspicion for ectopic pregnancy. The absence of an ectopic pregnancy on the USS does not exclude one.

First trimester

There is usually a history of PV bleeding and lower abdominal pain, although an empty gestational sac (or fetal pole with absent FH) may be an asymptomatic finding at booking scan. Miscarriage is inevitable if the internal cervical os is open or if products of conception (*not clots*) are passed. Rarely, products of one twin may be passed, with the other being viable, justifying USS in every case.

Management (when the os is closed) based on USS findings

Viable intrauterine pregnancy

Empty gestational sac Is this a true gestational sac (i.e. the sac has a double decidual ring) or a pseudo sac (suggestive of ectopic pregnancy)? If an empty gestational sac is greater than 25 mm maximum diameter the pregnancy is very likely to be non-viable (Fig. 5.1). This cannot be said with certainty, however, but if a pregnancy test was positive >3 weeks previously, the gestation will be at least 6 weeks' gestation and a fetal pole would always be seen on TV ultrasound. If the first positive pregnancy test was <3 weeks previously a conservative approach is most appropriate with a repeat scan in 10 days. Although this will add anxious waiting time for the patient, it is preferable to arranging an ERPOC on a viable pregnancy.

Pseudosac See Ectopic Pregnancy (p. 176) and Figure 5.2.

Fetal pole with no FH An FH is usually seen on TV scan if the fetal pole is >2–3 mm, but will always be seen by 6 mm (Fig. 5.3). A similar cut-off of 15 mm is appropriate for a TA scan. If in doubt, rescan 7–10 days later.

Empty uterus Either there has been a complete miscarriage (tissue may have been passed), the pregnancy is very early (e.g. <5 weeks), or there is an ectopic pregnancy. Ectopic pregnancy must be excluded. An intrauterine sac

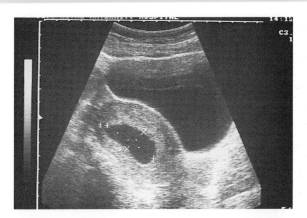

Fig. 5.1 Empty intrauterine gestational sac, 30 × 47 mm. Viability extremely unlikely.

will usually be seen on TV scan if the hCG is >1000 IU (>6500 IU for a TA scan), and its absence raises the possibility of an ectopic pregnancy. Serum levels of hCG should double in 48 hours if the pregnancy is viable and intrauterine; lower levels suggest an ectopic pregnancy (although by using this method in isolation 15% of intrauterine pregnancies would be diagnosed as ectopics and 13% of ectopics as intrauterine). If the level doubles and the patient remains well, repeat the USS in 1 week to ensure that the pregnancy is ongoing. If the hCG serum level is less than double, or steady, or only slightly reduced consider laparoscopy to exclude ectopic pregnancy.

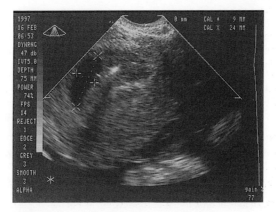

Fig. 5.2 Pseudosac with IUCD in situ. Ectopic pregnancy at laparoscopy.

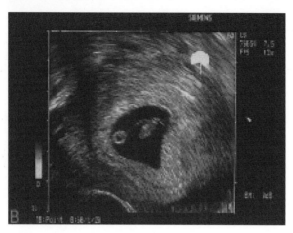

Fig. 5.3 Intrauterine gestational sac (note the double decidual ring) with a 5 mm fetal pole and yolk sac.

Retained products. Evacuation of retained products of conception (ERPOC) has become the established management for miscarriage with retained products. While this may still be offered there is evidence that if there is an incomplete miscarriage and the diameter of the retained products is <40 mm, ERPOC may not be necessary. The patient may be reviewed in 2 weeks and rescanned, at which time about 20% will still have retained products. This group may be offered ERPOC. All should be advised to return before 2 weeks if there is heavy bleeding, pain or fever.

Adnexal mass or ectopic pregnancy In ectopic pregnancy adnexal findings are of a sac (30%), a sac containing a yolk sac (15%) and a sac with a fetal pole and FH (15%). The absence of adnexal findings on USS therefore *does not exclude* an ectopic pregnancy. Ovarian cysts up to 3 cm in size are likely to be physiological and no further action is required. (Lancet 1995;345:86).

Second trimester
If there is no FH and no uterine activity use mifepristone and Cervagem. A history of painless cervical dilatation may indicate cervical incompetence.

After the miscarriage
All products of conception should be sent for histology to exclude gestational trophoblastic disease. There has been a bereavement and the parents have lost 'a baby'. They should be reassured that they did nothing which might have caused the miscarriage and given time to grieve. There is no medical indication for the woman to wait until trying to conceive again, but the couple may require contraception to allow time to grieve. There is often further upset around the EDD. The Miscarriage Association's telephone number is 01924 200799.

Septic abortion

This is rare (?? criminal interference). There is usually temperature >38°C, tachycardia, malaise, abdominal pain, marked tenderness and purulent vaginal loss. Endotoxic shock may develop (see p. 104). Usual organisms are Gram-negative bacteria, streptococci (haemolytic and anaerobic) and other anaerobes (e.g. bacteriodes).

RECURRENT SPONTANEOUS ABORTION (MISCARRIAGE)

The WHO definition is the consecutive loss of three or more fetuses weighing <500 g (incidence 0.5–1%). Those who have had three consecutive miscarriages still have a 70% chance of a normal outcome in their next pregnancy.

Investigation of recurrent miscarriage

- Check karyotype from both parents.
- Karyotype fetal products.
- Send maternal blood for lupus anticoagulant and anticardiolipin antibodies.
- Consider hysterosalpingogram and/or pelvic ultrasound (uterus and ovaries).

Causes and management

Antiphospholipid syndrome (≈15%) Miscarriage is more likely to occur in the presence of lupus anticoagulant and raised anticardiolipin antibodies (see p. 111).

Chromosomal abnormality (≈5%) This is usually a balanced reciprocal or Robertsonian translocation, and the finding of such an abnormality should prompt genetic referral (see also p. 9).

Cervical incompetence This is often diagnosed as a cause of midtrimester miscarriage, and cervical cerclage should probably only be considered when the miscarriage has been preceded by spontaneous rupture of membranes or painless cervical dilatation. The MRC/RCOG trial of cervical cerclage use demonstrated only a small decrease in preterm birth, but no survival improvement (Br J Obstet Gynaecol 1993:516). It should be noted, however, that entry criteria to this trial was for those in whom there was clinical doubt as to whether a suture was appropriate. Transabdominal cerclage has also been used (Eur J Obstet Gynaecol 1997:127), but is not without risk and should be considered a subspecialist procedure.

Thrombophilic defects

Retrospective studies have indicated an increased incidence of thrombophilic defects in those with recurrent miscarriage (activated protein C resistance, antithrombin III, protein C and protein S deficiency ± hyperhomocystinaemia). Evidence for the efficacy of treatment in this group is lacking (see also p. 111).

Anatomical uterine abnormality

- Congenital abnormalities, see p. 175.
- Fibroids: of uncertain significance, but large fibroids may be a cause of infertility and possibly miscarriage.

It is very difficult to estimate the significance of anatomical abnormalities and great caution is required before undertaking significant surgical procedures.

Other Although inadequate luteal support may be a cause of miscarriage, there has been no proven benefit from the use of progestogens or hCG. A higher LH level, as in PCOS, is also associated with recurrent miscarriage, but no effective treatment is known. It is also possible that mothers who share a high proportion of HLA antibodies with their partner fail to produce sufficient 'immune blocking antibodies' to protect the fetus from the mother's immune system. Injecting the mother with paternal white cells has not been shown to be effective. Miscarriage is also more likely in association with medical disorders (e.g. renal failure, thyroid dysfunction), although investigation for these is almost always normal.

CHRONIC PELVIC PAIN

Symptoms, clinical findings and laparoscopic findings correlate poorly and ≈50% of those who are laparoscoped show no abnormality. Of those with pelvic pain, ≈50% show significant emotional disturbance, but studies have also shown that pain itself may lead to neuroticism. A history of pelvic pain is associated with increased anxiety, an increased number of sexual partners and an increased incidence of psychosexual trauma, either as a child or later in life (Br J Obstet Gynaecol 1998:8).

Investigations

First admission for pain
Consider the possible causes (*Table 5.1*), check a pregnancy test, send swabs for infection (see p. 186) and arrange a USS (chlamydia screening can be carried out easily on first-void urines if PCR/LCR is available). If investigations are negative and the patient is improving, adopt a conservative approach. If becoming worse, consider laparoscopy.

TABLE 5.1	Causes of lower abdominal pain	
Gynaecological	Gastrointestinal	Urinary tract
PID (see p. 186)	Appendicitis	Recurrent or chronic infection
Ovarian cysts	Constipation	Calculus
Endometriosis (see p. 178)	Diverticular disease	
Adenomyosis	Irritable bowel syndrome	

Second admission for pain Consider laparoscopy, ideally on a routine list the following day, or as an outpatient. Treat significant pathology if identified.

After laparoscopy (if no pathology is identified) Reassure and *review again in the outpatient clinic* (if discharged without follow-up many will return with continuing pain). At review, many will be improved. If there are still problems retake the history, exploring psychological and psychosexual aspects if possible. Call a halt to investigations if the history is not suggestive of GI or GU pathology. If symptoms are suggestive of irritable bowel syndrome, consider a trial of Colofac tablets.   Mebeverine (anti muscarinic)

Management

- If adhesions have been found adhesiolysis may be considered, but there are no proven benefits from controlled studies.
- Consider a 3 month trial of ovarian suppression. The COC may help, but may not suppress ovarian function completely. GnRH agonists are an expensive treatment option and carry the risk of hypo-oestrogenic side-effects. Provera 30 mg/day is probably more appropriate.

   Reduction of symptoms following ovarian suppression suggests a genuine gynaecological cause. This syndrome of pain has been suggested by some to be due to 'pelvic venous congestion' (Lancet 1984:946), a syndrome characterized by lower abdominal pain, postcoital ache and ovaries tender to palpation.

- TAH and BSO is unlikely to be successful if there has been no improvement with ovarian suppression. Stovall et al (Obstet Gynecol 1990:326) reported on 99 women undergoing hysterectomy for chronic pelvic pain: 35% had adenomyosis or fibroids; 78% were improved after 1 year; and 22% had persistent pain.
- Refer to a psychologist if there is a high somatization score or history of sexual abuse.
- Consider complementary therapies.

CONTRACEPTION

> The 'failure rate' in the absence of any contraception (i.e. the fecundity rate) is 80–90:100 woman-years.

NATURAL METHODS

During the fertile period cervical mucus is clear, watery (i.e. of low viscosity) and is easily stretched into strands (Spinnbarkeit). In the non-fertile period it is viscous. This knowledge, used in combination with a midcycle core temperature rise (0.5–1°C) and awareness that the fertile period is 6 days before to 2 days after ovulation, has a failure rate in *well-motivated couples* of 2.8:100 woman years (Br Med J 1993:723). Full unsupplemented breast-feeding in which the mother is amenorrheoic is 98% effective in the first 6 months. Another method should be introduced if menses occur (bleeding before 56 days can be ignored), or with the introduction of supplementary foods, or after 6 months.

IUCD

The main mechanism of action of the IUCD is the reduction in the number of viable gametes, particularly sperm but also oocytes. The classification is outlined in Table 5.2.

TABLE 5.2 Classification of IUCDs (Fig. 5.4)

	Coil*	Failure rate	Lasts for
2nd generation	Multiload Cu250	1–2/100	3–5 years
	Nova T (Novagard)	1–2/100	
3rd generation	Multiload Cu375	0.5–1/100	≥5 years
	Copper Cu380 (slimline)	0.3–1/100	
4th generation	Gynefix frameless IUCD	0.5–1/100	5 years
Hormone-releasing intrauterine system	Levonorgestrel impregnated (releasing 20 µg/day). Systemic side effects (e.g. acne) are rare. See also Menorrhagia, p. 202		

*The number refers to the surface area of copper in mm^2.

Benefits
The IUCD is a highly effective method of contraception with virtually no systemic side-effects, and so it can be used by breast-feeding mothers.

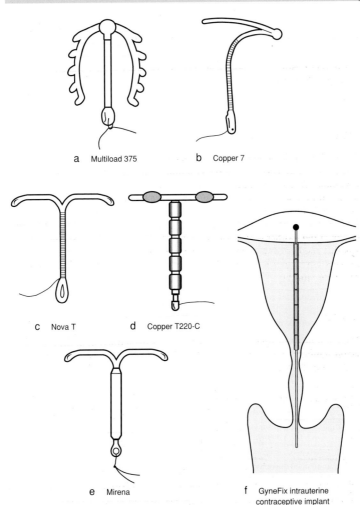

Fig. 5.4 Intrauterine contraceptive devices.

Side-effects

There may be some dysmenorrhoea, and bleeding is increased by an average of 40% (but much reduced with the levonorgestrel IUCD). The risk of ectopic pregnancy is reduced overall, but if pregnancy does occur it is more likely to be ectopic than if the IUCD was not present. The risk of PID is small and limited only to the first few weeks after insertion. Mild infection can be treated with the IUCD in situ, but if the device is removed because of infection it should not be re-inserted for 6 months. Asymptomatic actinomycoses on a smear test does not require treatment, but if there is any tenderness on VE, remove the IUCD and treat with high-dose penicillin for several weeks.

Contraindications

These include previous tubal pregnancy and PID. (If the patient is symptom free, and the PID was not severe, occurred >6 months previously and has not subsequently recurred, then this may be only a relative contraindication.) The use of IUCDs is also contraindicated in pregnancy, the immunosuppressed, those with a distorted uterine cavity, Wilson's disease or a past history of bacterial endocarditis or prosthetic valve replacement. It is relatively contraindicated with HIV infection.

Insertion

This requires training. Ideally, IUCDs should be inserted between days 1 and 7 of the cycle (earlier carries a higher expulsion rate, later and there may already be a viable pregnancy). They may also be inserted at the time of TOP (although the expulsion rate is higher) or 6 weeks postpartum (see also p. 168). Perform a speculum and pelvic examination, looking particularly for the position of the uterus, its size and the presence of fibroids. Under speculum visualization, and ideally in lithotomy, pass a sound to determine the length of the uterus and then place the IUCD at the fundus (it may be necessary to grasp the cervix with a Vulsellum or Rampley's sponge-holding forceps). Cut the threads to 3 cm and arrange for follow-up at 1 and 6 weeks to check the threads. The technique for inserting Gynefix is different, as the knot in the string needs to be embedded in the fundus; insertion is simple but requires appropriate training.

Lost thread

Arrange an USS to confirm that the IUCD has not been expelled and that it is still inside the uterine cavity. Insert a thread retrieval hook to try and bring the threads down. If this is not successful, remove the device with sponge-holding forceps, usually under GA. Hysteroscopy may be of help. If the coil is in the abdominal cavity, it should be sought and removed as it may lead to intense inflammatory reactions. Although inert devices (e.g. SAF-T coil and Lippes Loop) are no longer available, some women may still have them in situ and they may be deeply embedded.

Pregnancy

More than 90% of pregnancies are intrauterine. The problem with leaving an IUCD in situ is the increased risk of second trimester abortion (up to 50%) and later problems from APH, SB and preterm delivery. The coil should be removed in the first trimester, as this carries a lower overall risk. Do not attempt thread retrieval if the threads have been drawn up, but treat as a 'high-risk' pregnancy.

Removal
Start alternative methods of contraception before removal. The IUCD should be changed every 3–5 years (see Table 5.2) unless the woman is aged ≥40 years when the device is inserted, in which cause she can keep it until 1 year after her last menstrual period (i.e. menopause). The coil should ideally be left in situ after sterilization until after the next menstrual period.

ORAL CONTRACEPTIVES

Combined oral contraceptive (Table 5.3)
This acts mainly by inhibiting ovulation. The failure rate is 0.1–3:100 woman-years (although the higher incidence quoted includes some non-compliance). The tablets are taken daily for 21 days followed by a 7 day break during which there is a withdrawal bleed. It should be started on the first day of the cycle, or 3 weeks postpartum, or on the same day as an abortion or miscarriage.

Benefits
Oral contraceptives are very effective means of reversible contraception. They reduce blood loss and decrease the incidence of dysmenorrhoea, fibroids, ectopic pregnancy, endometriosis, functional ovarian cysts, ovarian cancer (by 40%), endometrial cancer (by 50%) and PID (due to increased mucus viscosity).

Side-effects
These are weight gain, breast tenderness, changes in libido, and an increase in the incidence of MI, stroke and venous thromboembolic disease (WHO Tech Rep Ser 887, 1998).

- The risk of MI is not increased in pill users who do not smoke and who do not have either hypertension or diabetes, regardless of age. Hypertension increases the risk threefold and smoking increases the risk tenfold in COC users.
- The risk of ischaemic stroke is increased by 1.5 at all ages, but that of haemorrhagic stroke is not increased until >35 years. Hypertension increases the risk of both (three- and tenfold, respectively) and smoking increases the risk threefold over that of non-users.
- The risk of venous thromboembolic disease is increased three- to sixfold in pill users over non-users and is unrelated to oestrogen if the dose is <50 μg ethinyloestradiol. Risks are unrelated to smoking or hypertension. Pills containing desogestrel and gestodene probably carry a small risk of venous thromboembolic disease above pills containing levonorgestrel. Desogestrel and gestodene were originally used because of their favourable effects on serum markers for cardiovascular and cerebrovascular disease, but there are insufficient data to show whether these benefits translate into a

genuine clinical benefit (Arch Intern Med 1997:1522). It is therefore advised that they should not be used by women with risk factors for thromboembolism including BMI >30 kg/m², varicose veins, immobility or family history of thrombosis (Br Med J 1995:1111).

TABLE 5.3   Classification of combined oral contraceptives

Ethinyloestradiol	Pill	Progestogen	Dose (mg)	Notes
20 µg	Mercilon	Desogestrel	0.15	Particularly suitable for the obese or older woman. Desogestrel has been reported to lead to better cycle control than
	Loestrin 20	Norethisterone	1	norethisterone
30 µg	Marvelon	Desogestrel	0.15	Desogestrel and gestodene may have
	Femodene (± ED) Minulet	Gestodene	0.075	less adverse effects on lipids than ethynodiol, levonorgestrel and norethisterone. There may, however, be an increased risk of venous thromboembolism (see text)
	Microgynon 30 (± ED) Ovranette	Levonorgestrel	0.15	
	Eugynon 30 Ovran 30	Levonorgestrel	0.25	
	Loestrin 30	Norethisterone	1.5	
35 µg	Brevinor Ovysmen	Norethisterone	0.5	
	Norimin	Norethisterone	1	
	Cilest	Norgestimate	0.25	Norgestimate may have less adverse effects on lipids than norethisterone, but probably has similar effects on venous thromboembolic disease as gestodene
50 µg	Ovran Norinyl-1	Levonorgestrel Norethisterone	0.25 1	For circumstances with reduced bio-availability, e.g. while using enzyme-inducing drugs. There is an increased possibility of side-effects

TABLE 5.4 Classification of progestogen only contraceptives		
Progestogen	Pill	Dose (mg)
Norethisterone type	Micronor	0.35
	Noriday	0.35
	Femulen	0.5
Levonorgestrel	Microval	0.03
	Norgeston	0.03
	Neogest	0.075

- The relative risk of breast cancer with COC users is 1.24, but there is a decreased risk of metastases (RR = 0.8). The relationship between the pill and breast cancer, therefore, remains unclear (increased detection or actual effect?).

Overall, COC use does not increase or decrease mortality – there is a lower death rate from ovarian carcinoma and a higher rate of mortality from circulatory disorders and cervical carcinoma. These effects are seen with those taking the pill and in the 10 years afterwards (Br Med J 1999;318:96).

Contraindications

These include pregnancy, severe or multiple risk factors for arterial disease, a history of arterial or venous thrombosis, IHD, severe hypertension, focal migraine, severe migraine, crescendo migraine, TIA, liver disorders, breast or genital tract carcinoma, history of HUS, or during pregnancy of pemphygoid gestationis, pruritus, chorea or cholestatic jaundice. The COC should not be taken by breast-feeding mothers as it interferes with lactation. Death due to the pill in those >35 years old is 8 times more common in those women who smoke, and either the pill or the smoking should be stopped at this age. Low-risk non-smokers may continue the COC until the menopause (although they will not know when this is without stopping it!).

Management

Check ups The woman should be seen usually at 3 months and thereafter every 6 months to have a BP check, discuss side-effects and ensure that she is up to date with her cervical smears. The objective is to achieve good cycle control with the lowest possible dose of oestrogen.

Breakthrough bleeding

This may take up to 6 months to resolve after starting a COC. It is uncertain whether this represents an increased risk of failure. Check compliance, a pregnancy test and exclude cervical pathology by speculum examination. Take a drug history (see Effectiveness, below). Then change to a pill with an increased dose of oestrogen, or return to an older Gestogen, or try a phasic pill.

Forgotten pill The pill should be taken as soon as it is remembered, and the next one again at the normal time. If the pill is taken more than 12 hours late, additional contraceptive methods are required for the next 7 days (e.g. condom). If these 7 days run past the end of the packet, the next packet should be started at once without leaving a gap. (If 'every day' (ED) pills are being used, the woman should miss out the seven inactive pills.) *The most critical time for missing pills is at the start of a packet (i.e. lengthening the pill-free interval).* If two or more pills are missed in the first 7 days, consider PCC.

Effectiveness This is reduced by liver enzyme inducers (most anticonvulsants, griseofulvin and rifampicin); therefore use a 50 µg ethinyloestradiol preparation. Vomiting and use of antibiotics may interfere with absorption, and additional precautions should be used for 7 days. Diarrhoea alone is not a significant problem.

The progestogen only pill (Table 5.4)
The failure rate is 0.3–4:100 woman-years. The pill is taken every day as close to the same time as possible (within a 3 hour window) and it acts on cervical mucus and alters the endometrium. The Gestogen dose is lower than in the COC and there is no oestrogen. Ovulation is inhibited in only ≈50%, and 20–25% have functional ovarian cysts (usually asymptomatic). The main side-effect is irregular bleeding, or occasionally, amenorrhoea. The overall ectopic risk is reduced, but if pregnancy does occur it is more likely to be an ectopic than if the POP was not being taken. Unlike the COC, it is not contraindicated in breast-feeding and may be used in those with diabetes, hypertension and smokers >35 years old. Side-effects include nausea, vomiting, headache, breast discomfort, depression, skin disorders and weight changes. There is no significant increase in the risk of venous thromboembolic disease. (For the different types of pill available, see Table 5.4.)

If a pill is missed, it should be taken as soon as it is remembered, and the next one taken at its usual time. If the pill was more than 3 hours overdue, additional protection should be used for the next 7 days. Vomiting may interfere with absorption, so that additional precautions should again be used for 7 days.

EMERGENCY CONTRACEPTION

The Yuzpe method is the most commonly used in the UK. It should be used with caution in those with a history of venous thromboembolic disease and, it is not suitable for those with focal migraine at the time of presentation. It involves taking two tablets, each with ethinyl oestradiol 50 µg and levonorgestrel 250 µg (e.g. Schering PC4 or Ovran) followed by a further two tablets 12 hours later. If tablets are vomited, an extra two should be taken. The pills inhibit or delay ovulation, can be used up to 72 hours after intercourse and prevent 75% of pregnancies which would have occurred that.

cycle. It is more successful the earlier it is taken (Lancet 1998;332:428). The next 'period' may be early, on time or late, and barrier contraception should be used until then. If there has been no 'period' after 3–4 weeks, a pregnancy test must be arranged (pregnancy after postcoital contraception is *not* in itself an indication for TOP as there have been no reported teratogenic problems). An IUCD can be inserted up to 5 days after the estimated day of ovulation (which may be >5 days after intercourse) and has an almost 100% success rate in preventing pregnancy that cycle. Levonorgestrel alone (0.75 mg twice, separated by 12 hours) may be more effective and has fewer side-effects than the Yuzpe method. This may be marketed in the UK in the near future.

INJECTABLE PROGESTOGENS

These carry a failure rate of 0–1:100 woman years. Depo Provera (150 mg medroxyprogesterone acetate IM 12 weekly) is commonly used. 80% of women will be amenorrhoeic by 1 year, although 2% will develop troublesome menorrhagia. As heavy bleeding can occur, Depo Provera is best left until 6 weeks postpartum, using other methods from 3 to 6 weeks, although Oenanthe may be given immediately postpartum. Delayed return to fertility may occur, lasting up to 18 months. Most women gain some weight. Recent studies suggest that the effect on reduced bone mineral density is unlikely to be clinically significant, but concerns remain about its use in adolescents who have yet to reach their peak bone mass. It should also perhaps be discontinued in those >45 years old for the same reason.

INJECTABLES

Norplant has now been withdrawn from the UK market. It has a failure rate of 0–1:100 woman-years and consisted of six subdermal capsules (each the size of a matchstick) inserted SC under local anaesthetic. They lasted 5 years. Irregular and often frequent bleeding occurred in 70% of cases, and did not really improve with time. Ovulation occurred in about 10%. Training was required for the removal of the capsules.

Implanon has just been launched in the UK. A single rod with a disposable inserter, it contains desogestrel alone at a dose that inhibits ovulation in all users, so that more women would have amenorrhoea than had it with Norplant. It lasts 3 years.

BARRIER METHODS

These reduce the transmission of most STDs with both vaginal and anal intercourse.

Condoms These are effective when used properly and with spermicidal cream. The risk of bursting is reduced if air is expelled from the teat (failure rate 2–15:100 woman-years). Manufacturers are now producing different sizes, which may help with recurrent bursting.

Diaphragms These stretch from the posterior fornix to above the symphysis pubis (like ring pessaries) whereas cervical caps fit over the cervix (which needs to be prominent). They should be used with spermicide, inserted <2 hours before intercourse and removed at least 6 hours later. Side-effects include UTIs and problems with rubber hypersensitivity (failure rate 2–15:100 woman-years). A new silicone cervical cap may come onto the UK market soon, and would be an option for women with latex allergy.

Female condoms These condoms (e.g. Femidom) have a high failure rate, usually due to the penis being inserted between the condom and the vaginal wall.

STERILIZATION

Consider which partner should be sterilized. How stable is the relationship? If the woman is obese, it may be technically difficult to undertake laparoscopy. Are there concerns about masculinity or femininity? Might a hysterectomy be better if there is significant menstrual dysfunction or history of CIN? Legally, consent is only required from the person wishing to be sterilized. Preoperative counselling details are outlined below and *these details must be recorded in the notes*:

- Irreversibility and alternative methods of contraception (10% regret their decision at 18 months and 1% seek reversal, especially those who are single and younger).
- Failure rates and, in women, the risk of ectopic pregnancy.
- A woman should be aware that if laparoscopy is unsuccessful or if there are complications, it might be necessary to perform a laparotomy under the same GA.
- After sterilization in men, it is necessary to wait until two clear semen specimens have been obtained (months) before other contraception is stopped. In women, it is necessary to continue with alternative contraception until the next menstrual period.

Female sterilization

This is usually carried out laparoscopically by tubal occlusion (Falope rings, Hulka clips, Filshie clips or diathermy) but can be performed by laparotomy, at caesarean section or, more radically, by hysterectomy. For laparoscopy, clips are considered by some to have the lowest failure rate (RCOG Clinical Guideline 4, 1999), although other evidence suggests a higher failure rate for clips (Table 5.5). Failure rates are particularly high in very young women.

Tubal occlusion after the age of 30 is not associated with an increase in abdominal pain, dyspareunia or menstrual disturbance; there is debate about this possibility before this age, although it is possible that menstrual disturbance has been masked by the COC prior to the operation.

TABLE 5.5   The 10 year failure rate following tubal sterilization from the CREST study (Am J Obstet Gynecol 1996:1161)

Method	10 year probability of pregnancy (per 1000 procedures)
Bipolar coagulation	24.8
Unipolar coagulation	7.5
Silicone rubber band application	17.7
Spring-clip application	36.5
Interval partial salpingectomy	20.1
Postpartum salpingectomy	7.5
All methods	18.5

Male sterilization

Vasectomy can be performed on an outpatient basis under local anaesthesia. Bruising and haematoma formation are not uncommon. The failure rate is 1:1000 following two negative semen samples. The evidence suggests that the incidence of testicular cancer is not increased, although there is still some concern about the risk of prostate cancer.

DEVELOPMENTAL PROBLEMS

DELAYED PUBERTY AND PRIMARY AMENORRHOEA

In normal development there is thought to be some form of trigger which leads to pulsatile release of LH and FSH between the ages of 5 and 10 years, with an ovarian response occurring usually after the age of 8 years. The first sign of puberty in girls is increased growth and, almost simultaneously, breast budding followed by the appearance of pubic hair. Menarche usually follows within 2 years of the first breast and hair development, always after, and usually within, 1 year of the peak growth velocity. Although deviation from this sequence (loss of consonance) is 'abnormal', it may occur in up to 50% of girls. Primary amenorrhoea is defined as no menstruation by the age of 14 years accompanied by failure to develop secondary sexual characteristics. It is also defined as no menstruation by the age of 16 years with normal sexual development.

Initial management

- Exclude pregnancy.
- Ask about chronic illnesses, anorexia, excessive fitness training or a family history of delayed puberty. Also ask about heart problems (associated with chromosomal disorders), urinary or bowel problems (associated with anatomical abnormalities of the genital tract), hernia repairs (gonadal disorder) and general development (slow in hypothyroidism).
- Carry out an examination, especially height and weight, the presence of secondary sexual characteristics, hirsutism, virilization and visual fields (a vaginal examination should only be considered in sexually active girls). Look for signs of dysharmonious development (e.g. pubic hair but no breast development) and for stigmata of Turner's syndrome.
- Serum for LH and FSH (low with constitutional delay), testosterone (increased in polycystic ovarian syndrome), free T_4, TSH (increased in primary hypothyroidism) and Prl (the patient should ideally be unstressed for Prl levels).
- Consider a karyotype.
- Consider obtaining an X-ray for bone age if constitutional delay is suspected.
- Consider giving 17-hydroxyprogesterone if development is dysharmonious. Also, consider a pelvic USS and skull radiograph.

Causes and further management

Normal secondary sexual characteristics but primary amenorhoea

This is most commonly caused by an imperforate hymen and is characterized by cyclical pain and a haematocolpos. A cruciate incision, usually under anaesthesia, is all that is required. Much more rarely, there is a horizontal septae or an absent uterus (see p. 174). A progesterone challenge test will identify constitutional menstrual delay (i.e. will result in bleeding only if the oestradiol level and genital tract is normal). Give Provera 10 mg TID PO for 10 days, or gestone 100–200 mg IM stat. There should be a withdrawal bleed within 10–14 days of the injection or 10–14 days after stopping the oral progestogen.

Poor or absent secondary sexual characteristics

Constitutional delay The diagnosis is likely in a healthy adolescent who is short for the family but appropriate for the stage of puberty and bone age. There is often a family history and it may be associated with chronic systemic disease (rare, but consider decreased T_4 and malabsorption). If the X-ray bone age is less than the chronological age then it is reasonable to adopt a conservative approach. Anorexia nervosa should also be considered.

Ovarian dysfunction This may be due to gonadal agenesis with Turner's syndrome (see p. 9) or Turner's mosaic. Treatment is specialized, as oestrogen treatment may predispose to short stature by premature epiphyseal closure. Therapy is with ethinyloestradiol, initially 1–2 µg/day PO increasing to 10 µg/day over the next 18 months. A progestogen (e.g. Norethisterone 350 µg/day) is then added for 5 days every 4 weeks. The dose of oestrogen is increased to 20–30 µg/day and the COC substituted. The polycystic ovarian syndrome (see p. 182) may occasionally present as primary amenorrhoea.

Hypothalamopituitary disorders Hypogonadotrophic hypogonadism is usually associated with pituitary tumours and other pituitary deficiencies. In Kallmann syndrome there is a congenital deficiency of LHRH and absent olfactory sensation. Hypothyroidism is likely to cause pubertal delay. Hyperprolactinaemia is rare.

INTERSEX DISORDERS AND AMBIGUOUS GENITALIA

> Early multidisciplinary subspecialist involvement is essential, particularly surrounding the issues of genital surgery and gender assignment. There will be initial shock at the diagnosis, with possible subsequent depression, doubts of gender, concerns over fertility, issues of sexuality, cultural problems and a sense of worthlessness. Peer support from those with similar problems is essential.

In those with XY chromosomes, testosterone masculinizes the otherwise female external genitalia and stimulates the mesonephric (Wolffian) system to develop. Mullerian inhibitory factor inhibits the paramesonephric (Mullerian) system, which would otherwise form female internal genitalia.

XY but look female (male pseudohermaphroditism)

Testicular feminization syndrome (androgen insensitivity) This is an XL recessive disorder due to the absence of androgen receptors. There are complete and incomplete forms. Presentation is usually after puberty, with amenorrhoea in the presence of normal breast development, scanty pubic and axillary hair, a blind-ending vagina, absent uterus, and female habitus and psychosexual orientation. Gonadectomy is essential because of the risk of malignant change; this should probably be done before puberty and followed by an exogenous hormone puberty induction.

5α-reductase deficiency
There is an AR target enzyme defect. At puberty, considerable, but still incomplete, virilization occurs, with male body habitus, psychosexual orientation and gender conversion.

Failure of testicular development This may occur with true gonadal agenesis. The internal and external genitalia are female. This is rare.

XX but look male (female pseudohermaphroditism)

Congenital adrenal hyperplasia This accounts for 70% of ambiguous genitalia. There is an AR enzyme defect in aldosterone synthesis which leads to an increase in androgens. In the commonest form, 21-hydroxylase deficiency, two-thirds have a salt-losing crisis, often within the first 4 weeks of life, which requires long-term mineralocorticoid replacement. There are ambiguous genitalia which may require a reduction clitoroplasty, although there is an argument against such a procedure as future sexual sensation may be reduced. The subsequent pregnancy rate in non-salt-losers is 60%, but only around 2% in salt-losers themselves. Diagnosis is by demonstrating an elevated serum 17-hydroxyprogesterone level or an increase in pregnanetriol and adrenal androgen metabolites in urine. 11-hydroxylase deficiency and 3α-hydroxysteroid dehydrogenase deficiency are rarer forms (see also p. 27). In those couples known to be heterozygotes for the genes (i.e. previously affected children) it may be reasonable to start dexamethasone 0.2 mg/kg/day from before 8 weeks' gestation, carry out a CVS and continue treatment if the fetus is female and is homozygous. Concerns have been raised about a possible steroid effect on later intellectual function.

Exogenous administration of androgens In pregnancy, the exogenous administration of androgens (e.g. Danazol) may lead to virilization of a female fetus.

Other rare abnormalities

These may occur with XO, XX or XY chimerism. True hermaphroditism (i.e. the presence of male and female gonadal tissue) is also rare.

ABNORMAL GENITAL TRACT DEVELOPMENT

Vagina

 Early multidisciplinary subspecialist involvement is essential.

There may be horizontal septae, vertical septae, or the vagina may be absent.

Horizontal septae There may be cryptomenorrhoea with cyclical pain and a haematocolpos. If obstruction is caused simply by the hymen (blood looks blue behind it), then a cruciate incision, usually under anaesthesia, is all that is required. If there is a horizontal septum secondary to a vertical fusion defect (looks pink rather than blue) the situation is potentially more serious and should be referred to a specialist surgeon. If the septum is in the low or midportion of the vagina, *total* excision and resuturing is necessary. If the septum is high, a combined abdominal and vaginal approach may be required. Pregnancy rates are excellent with low septae (consider later endometriosis), but are only around 25% for those higher in the vagina.

Vertical septae These are caused by horizontal fusion defects and may be associated with abnormal uterine development. Although presentation may be with dyspareunia, infertility or, occasionally, in advanced labour, the septum may be asymptomatic. The septum can be thick, and good pedicles should be taken during removal as there is a tendency for them to retract.

Vaginal atresia This is associated with an absent, or only a rudimentary, uterus and is known as the Rokitansky syndrome. Presentation is at puberty with amenorrhoea (or cryptomenorrhoea) in the presence of normal secondary sexual characteristics. If the uterus is non-functioning it is possible to create a vagina with regular use of vaginal dilators, or by one of a variety of surgical techniques. Surrogacy is an option (risk of recurrence in these offspring is probably small).

Uterus
Abnormal uterine shapes are usually asymptomatic but may present with primary infertility, recurrent pregnancy loss or menstrual dysfunction (oligomenorrhoea, dysmenorrhoea, menorrhagia). In pregnancy, there may be preterm labour or abnormal fetal lie.

Unicornuate uterus With this there is a particularly high miscarriage rate and a pregnancy developing in a rudimentary horn may lead to rupture and haemorrhage. If the abnormality is detected the rudimentary horn should be removed electively, either prior to conception or in early pregnancy if the embryo is confirmed to be in that horn.

Bicornuate uterus This may carry a pregnancy to an adequately advanced gestation, and this chance probably increases with subsequent pregnancies. A 'Strassman' procedure will correct the defect, but the benefits for pregnancy are unproven.

Septum of a septate uterus This is best removed hysteroscopically.

PRE-PUBERTAL PROBLEMS

See also Primary Amenorrhoea (p. 171) and Ambiguous Genitalia (p. 173).

Vaginal discharge
Such a symptom raises the possibility of, but does not necessarily imply, sexual abuse.

- Non-microbial causes. Threadworms are possible. Foreign-body insertion is rare.
- Microbial causes. Investigation is difficult to interpret as there are little data on the commensal profile of children. In those with discharge, the GpA streptococcus is commonly found, followed by *H. influenzae* and candida. Bowel flora are also common. Gardnerella and *Trichomonas vaginalis* are probably not commensals. Swabs should also be checked for *Chlamydia* and *N. gonorrhoea*.

Sexual abuse

 There are numerous pitfalls to the clinical examination, and you may be expected to demonstrate a depth of experience in court which you do not actually have. Early senior multidisciplinary help is essential in this highly emotive area where incorrect interpretation of the signs may have major consequences. A colposcope is important and photographic records are extremely useful.

This is the involvement of dependent sexually immature children and adolescents in sexual activity they do not truly comprehend and to which they are unable to give informed consent and which violates social taboos or family roles. The abuser is usually male and well known to the child and family. It may present acutely, following injury or allegation, or may be suggested by precociousness, self-harming (usually in older children/teenagers, and may include drugs and prostitution), eating disorders, enuresis, encopresis, sleep problems, lowered achievements, psychosomatic problems and attention-seeking behaviour.

The history should be carefully taken and documented, and the social work team involved if appropriate. Examination, which usually does not require anaesthetic, should involve specialists and may include paediatricians and a police surgeon, particularly in the acute situation. Swabs (which may include swabs for DNA analysis) should be taken with a 'secure chain of evidence' in case required for a later legal action. Look for bleeding, bruising or any other area of injury particularly lacerations at the posterior fourchette and perineal abrasions. A normal hymen has a number of different shapes (annular, crescentic, fimbriated, septate, sleeve or funnel shaped). Notches and clefts can be highly suggestive of penetrating injury, but may be normal if associated with an intravaginal ridge above them; they are very rare in the posterior segment in non-abused girls. Straddle injuries very rarely affect the hymen, and there is much more likely to be bruising anterior to the vagina or laterally (e.g. labia majora). It is also rare for tampon use to cause hymenal injury (although it may increase the diameter slightly), and there are no reported cases of congenital absence of the hymen. A normal prepubertal hymen does not exclude abuse.

ECTOPIC PREGNANCY

This refers to any non-intrauterine pregnancy and, although the pregnancies may be ovarian, cervical or intra-abdominal, the vast majority are tubal. The incidence of tubal pregnancy is 1:200–400 pregnancies, with 50% occurring in the ampulla, 28% in the isthmus and the rest either fimbrial or interstitial. There may be a history of a previous ectopic pregnancy, previous surgery, PID, endometriosis, IVF, GIFT or ZIFT, but 50% occur in those with no predisposing risk factors.

Clinical features

Clinical features range from no symptoms at all, to right, left or bilateral lower abdominal pain, PV bleeding, intra-abdominal haemorrhage (peritonism and shoulder tip pain) and collapse. Pelvic examinations should be gentle to avoid tubal rupture. A positive pregnancy test in the absence of a demonstrable intrauterine pregnancy should always be considered to be an ectopic pregnancy until proven otherwise. Undiagnosed intra-abdominal pregnancies have progressed to term to be delivered by caesarean section (do not attempt to remove the placenta).

Investigations

Check a chlamydia swab. An USS scan is most useful in demonstrating an intrauterine pregnancy. A gestational sac may be confused with a pseudosac (due to thickened endometrium), which is seen in 20% of ectopic pregnancies and which lacks the echogenic ring of a gestational sac (see Figs 5.1–5.3). A true sac is usually smooth, eccentrically placed, has a double rim and may contain a yolk sac. Adnexal findings are of a sac (30%), a sac containing a yolk sac (15%) and a sac with a fetal pole and FH (15%). The absence of adnexal findings on USS therefore *does not exclude an ectopic pregnancy*.

Management

Management depends on the overall clinical picture, the scan result and the hCG:

- If the patient is collapsed, shocked and has a positive pregnancy test, set up *two* IV infusions and crossmatch 6 units of RCC. Infuse colloid, crystalloid and, afterwards, if necessary, O negative or uncrossmatched group-specific blood. Arrange theatre urgently.
- If there is a positive pregnancy test with clinical signs of an ectopic pregnancy (pelvic tenderness, cervical excitation, shoulder tip pain) and an empty uterus on TV ultrasound, carry out a diagnostic laparoscopy.
- If there is a positive pregnancy test, an empty uterus and no clinical signs, check a quantitative hCG. If >1000 IU following a TV scan or >6500 IU following a TA scan, consider laparoscopy. Otherwise, repeat after at least 48 hours, as above. If less than doubling, or steady, or only slightly reduced, consider laparoscopy to exclude ectopic pregnancy.
- If the hCG levels are falling rapidly, the pregnancy (whether an intrauterine or ectopic) is aborting. If the patient is well, conservative management is often appropriate, with further hCG checks to ensure that the level continues to fall. Laparoscopy may be warranted if symptoms develop.

Treatment

Surgical treatment may be carried out laparoscopically or at laparotomy. Laparotomy is preferred if there is significant haemodynamic compromise. Although laparoscopy has the advantage of shorter hospital stay and quicker recovery time over laparotomy, subsequent reproductive outcome is similar or possibly slightly better.

The surgery can be either by salpingectomy (removal of the tube) or salpingostomy (a linear incision is made over the ectopic using unipolar needlepoint diathermy, the ectopic removed, and the tube left to close spontaneously). Salpingostomy carries a similar, or possibly slightly better intrauterine pregnancy rate than salpingectomy, but higher subsequent ectopic rate of 15% vs 10% (Fertil Steril 1997:421). With a fimbrial ectopic it might also be possible to 'milk' the pregnancy from the tube at laparotomy. Salpingectomy is indicated in the presence of uncontrollable bleeding, recurrent ectopic in the same tube, a severely damaged tube, or when childbearing is complete. If the tube is conserved it is essential to ensure that the hCG is falling; if not, there is likely to be residual trophoblast. The hCG should fall to 25% of the pretreatment level within 4 days of surgery (average time to an undetectable level is 4 weeks).

There is growing interest in medical management of ectopic pregnancy, particularly with methotrexate (e.g. at a dose of $50 \, mg/m^2$ IM) without folate rescue, providing the patient is haemodynamically stable, any USS visualized ectopic is <3.5 cm and there are no blood or liver problems. (Note: Before initiating treatment, see the excellent and detailed protocol in Am J Obstet Gynecol 1993;168:1759).

ENDOMETRIOSIS

Endometriosis is present in 10–25% of women presenting with gynaecological symptoms. The commonest sites are the ovary (55%), posterior broad ligament (35%), anterior and posterior pouch of Douglas (34%) and uterosacral ligaments (28%). There is a great variation in symptoms, and there is poor correlation between symptoms and laparoscopic findings. Pain is usually associated with menstruation or may occur immediately premenstrually. Dyspareunia is common. There may rarely be rupture or torsion of an endometrioma, irregular menses or, rarely, cyclical problems with rectal bleeding, tenesmus, diarrhoea, constipation, haemoptysis, dysuria, ureteric colic or scar pains.

The chance of successful pregnancy may be as low as half that of the normal population. This may be due to an endocrinopathy, reduced frequency of coitus, tubal dysfunction, early pregnancy failure or reduced sperm function (secretions are luteolytic and the increased numbers of macrophages are highly phagocytic to sperm).

Laparoscopically, endometriosis may appear white or red (active lesions), as black/brown 'powder' burns or as white plaques of old collagen. There may also be circular defects in the peritoneum or endometriomas, with 'chocolate' fluid containing debris from cyclical menstruation.

Medical treatment principles

Drug treatment is not indicated for the treatment of asymptomatic, minimal or minor endometriosis in patients wishing to conceive. For symptomatic relief in such patients, treatment should be limited to 3 months. If treatment is required, the objective is to abolish menstruation. Recurrence after treatment is common.

All therapies suppress ovulation, and thus conception is unlikely with good compliance. Nonetheless, it is still advisable for patients to use barrier methods of contraception (unless using COC or GnRH analogues). To avoid inadvertent administration during pregnancy, all therapies should be initiated within the first 3 days of the start of a menstrual period.

- For symptomatic endometriosis, continuous progestogen therapy, e.g. medroxyprogesterone acetate (Provera) 10 mg TID for 90 days, is most cost-effective, has fewer side-effects and is more suitable for long-term use compared with more expensive alternatives. Another very cost-effective alternative suitable for longer term use is the continuous low-dose COC. Failure to suppress symptoms, troublesome and persistent breakthrough bleeding or problems with side-effects would be an indication for alternative therapy.
- Second-line drugs are the GnRH analogues, which can be administered by nasal spray or implants (e.g. nafarelin, buseralin, goseralin, leuproelin acetate) and the androgen Danazol (Danol) 200 mg once to three times daily. The costs are similar. Choice will depend on the side-effect profile; e.g. overweight women or those tending towards hirsutism would do better with a GnRH analogue. Underweight women or those particularly at risk of bone loss should be prescribed Danazol. Danazol is unlikely to be satisfactory for women already experiencing weight gain or bloating with a progestogen or the COC. Therapy for both should be restricted to 6 months (or less if fertility is desired).

Failure of symptom relief if amenorrhoea has been induced implies that the problem is unlikely to be due to endometriosis and is an indication for a review of the diagnosis. It is not necessary to achieve complete amenorrhoea if patients have a good symptomatic response, provided that spotting or bleeding is acceptable to the patient.

Surgical treatment

Conservative treatment This may be carried out at laparoscopy or laparotomy, and includes diathermy destruction or laser vaporization of endometriosis deposits. Surgical treatment of minimal and mild endometriosis improves fertility in subfertile women, and may have some fertility benefit in moderate/severe disease (medical treatment does not improve fertility in any form of endometriosis). Surgery for large endometriotic cysts may improve the outlook in IVF cycles.

Radical surgery (BSO ± TAH) This may be indicated for those in whom fertility is no longer required. HRT may lead to a recurrence of endometriosis in a small proportion, but should not be withheld if there are significant symptoms or long-term risk factors.

FIBROIDS

Fibroids occur in ≈20% of women in the reproductive years, particularly in the obese, those of low parity and those of negroid origin. There is a reduced frequency in smokers and those on COC. Fibroids are smooth muscle in origin (despite their name) and are often multiple. Although more than 50% are asymptomatic, they may lead to menorrhagia, subfertility, recurrent spontaneous abortion, urinary symptoms and, occasionally, pain. Pain is usually acute, due to degeneration, and is only occasionally chronic. Hyaline degeneration (the commonest) leads to a smoother and more homogeneous lesion which may become cystic if liquefaction occurs. Fatty change is rare. Calcification usually occurs in postmenopausal subserosal fibroids. Red degeneration presents almost exclusively in pregnancy with acute pain, fever and localized tenderness. The exact risk of sarcomatous change remains uncertain, but is probably <0.1%.

Types

Fibroids may be of four types (Fig. 5.5):

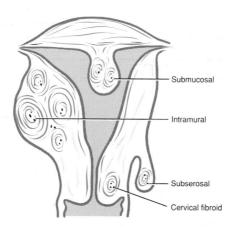

Submucosal

Intramural

Subserosal

Cervical fibroid

Fig. 5.5 Uterine fibroids.

Subserosal There is no restriction on growth and they may become very large, pedunculated (and torted) or even develop their own blood supply from the omentum. They may extend into the broad ligament or may arise separately from the round ligament.

Intramural There is a false capsule of connective tissue.

Submucous These are less common, are covered with endometrium, may be pedunculated and may prolapse through the cervix.

Cervical These may lead to ureteric and urethral obstruction. Surgery may be technically demanding due to the close proximity of the bladder and ureters.

Investigations

- Check a FBC in case menorrhagia has led to anaemia. There may very rarely be polycythaemia due to erythropoietin production (reversible after surgical removal).
- Carry out a clinical examination and an USS.

Treatment

- This should be conservative if the patient is asymptomatic. As the risk of sarcomatous change is probably <0.1% prophylactic removal is probably not justified. There is no evidence that absolute size or rate of increase in size are indicators of sarcomatous change.
- Of those women with a blood loss >200 ml, 50% have fibroids. The GnRH analogues, e.g. goseralin (Zoladex) 3.6 mg SC injection monthly, leuprorelin acetate (Prostap) 3.75 mg SC monthly, buseralin (Supracur) 300 µg (= 1 puff each nostril) TID intranasal spray or nafarelin (Synarel) 400 µg (= 1 puff each nostril) BD intranasally, will reduce the fibroid size (up to 50%, the greatest reduction occurring in the first 3 months of treatment). The effects are reversed on discontinuation of treatment. Their use for 2–3 months preoperatively in those awaiting surgery reduces blood loss at operation (Br J Obstet Gynaecol 1994:438).
- If there is infertility, or recurrent miscarriage, consider surgical treatment only as a last resort, either with hysteroscopic resection or myomectomy. As there are no supporting data for either, great caution is required before planning surgery. For the myomectomy, ideally use the 'hood' method of Bonney, closing the incision anteriorly to minimize posterior adhesions to the adnexa. There is a risk of heavy blood loss at surgery, which may necessitate hysterectomy. It is considered acceptable by some to undertake a vaginal delivery after myomectomy, but others would carry out a caesarean section irrespective of whether the uterine cavity was entered at operation or not. Pregnancy in the presence of fibroids carries a greater risk of miscarriage and preterm labour. Red degeneration is common, but mechanical difficulties are rare.

HIRSUTISM

> The definition is subjective, e.g. a patient saying 'I have too much hair'. It may also be defined as 'male-type body hair distribution'. Hirsutism is only rarely associated with virilization (clitoromegaly, breast atrophy, frontal baldness, deepening voice, muscle growth). Staging is according to the Ferriman–Gallwey chart.

Other causes include drugs (phenytoin, diazoxide), hypothyroidism and anorexia. The main causes of hirsutism are listed in Table 5.6.

TABLE 5.6	Causes of hirsutism			
Cause	Time to presentation	Virilization	Amenorrhoea/ oligomenorrhoea	Frequency
Idiopathic	Years	No	No	Common
PCOS	Years	No	Yes	Common
CAH	Years	Yes	Yes	Rare
Tumour	Months	Yes	Yes	Rare

Idiopathic hirsutism
This may be due to end-organ hypersensitivity. There may be a slight increase in testosterone and androsterone but the LH/FSH ratio is normal.

Polycystic ovarian syndrome (PCOS) (Br Med J 1998;317:329)
The diagnosis of PCOS is based on the presence of some or all of oligo- or amenorrhoea (present in 80%), anovulatory infertility (74%), hirsutism (69%), acne, central obesity (i.e. BMI >25) (49%), USS ovarian morphology, increased testosterone, increased free androgen index, and increased LH with normal FSH. As diagnostic criteria are not precise, incidences of 0.5–25% have been quoted. There is good evidence for the hypothesis that decreased peripheral insulin sensitivity (exacerbated by obesity) leads to hyperinsulinaemia; the increased insulin level then stimulates theca-cell androgen production and has an adverse effect on the lipid profile.

Treatment is symptomatic. The COC has been used to regulate menses but, while it reduces androgen levels, it exacerbates insulin resistance and may be relatively contraindicated in obese women. Hirsutism may be treated with the COC or cyproterone acetate (see p. 184), and clomiphene is useful for anovulatory infertility (see p. 196). Laparoscopic laser or diathermy to the ovary may also give short-term benefits for anovulation, but only when the patient is clomiphene resistant. The cornerstone to management, however, is weight reduction, which reduces insulin resistance, corrects the hormone imbalance and promotes ovulation. Recent work has been directed towards the use of insulin sensitizing agents (e.g. metformin) and, although trial numbers are small, this therapeutic option shows promise.

PCOS may be considered a systemic metabolic condition rather than one of primary gynaecological origin, and individuals may gain benefit from early screening for cardiovascular risk factors, particularly raised BP and glucose intolerance. Long term there is an increased risk of cardiovascular disease, NIDDM, endometrial hyperplasia and endometrial and breast carcinoma (there is no proven link with ovarian tumours).

Congenital adrenal hyperplasia (CAH)
See p. 174.

Tumours
These are very rare. Ovarian tumours are usually thecomas or Sertoli/Leydig cell tumours. Adrenal tumours are adenomas or adenocarcinomas.

Investigations
Serum testosterone, DHAS, 17-hydroxyprogesterone, early follicular LH/FSH, T_4, TSH, prolactin and USS of the ovaries.

- An early follicular phase LH/FSH ratio >3, with an elevated testosterone (>3 nmol/l) and the USS findings of multiple (>8) small, peripherally placed follicular ovarian cysts surrounding a thickened echodense stroma is considered diagnostic of PCOS.
- DHAS is 90% adrenal and is often elevated in PCOS (normal range 1.5–11.5 µmol/l). If normal, an adrenal tumour is very unlikely (although the level may be normal in late onset CAH).
- If 17-hydroxyprogesterone is elevated, arrange a short synacthen test. An excessive elevation of 17-hydroxyprogesterone confirms the diagnosis of CAH, and life-long dexamethasone treatment is required.
- If Cushing syndrome is suspected clinically, collect a 24-hour urinary cortisol and arrange a low-dose dexamethasone suppression test.

If the testosterone level is >7 nmol/l suspect an androgen secreting tumour and arrange an USS, CT or MRI scan to aid localization.

Treatment (Br J Obstet Gynaecol 1998:687)
Treatment of idiopathic or PCOS associated hirsutism takes at least 6 months to show significant improvement (for PCOS, see also p. 182):

- Weight loss (a BMI in the range 19–25 is ideal).
- Cosmetic procedures (e.g. electrolysis) are very useful. Shaving does *not* lead to thicker stubble or make hirsutism worse.
- The COC reduces ovarian androgen production and increases SHBG, thereby lowering the level of free testosterone. It may usefully contain cyproterone acetate (an antiandrogen with marked progestogenic activity), which reduces hirsutism markedly in some, but not all, patients (e.g. Dianette: cyproterone acetate 2 mg and ethinyloestradiol 35 µg).
- Cyproterone acetate may be more effectively used when taken along with a COC. Dianette may be used. Cyproterone 25–100 mg should be taken with the first 10 pills of each Dianette cycle. Following improvement, maintenance treatment may be continued with Dianette alone. There have been a small number of case reports of hepatotoxicity with prolonged high-dose cyproterone acetate, so LFTs should be checked.
- In occasional cases of PCOS with excess adrenal androgens, low-dose dexamethasone (e.g. 0.25 mg nocte) may be useful and may increase the chance of ovulation, but be aware of the additional risks of steroid therapy in often already obese patients.

HYPERPROLACTINAEMIA

Hyperprolactinaemia may be due to an adenoma (40–50%), secondary to other causes (rare) or idiopathic (the remainder). It may present as galactorrhoea, amenorrhoea or infertility and should be diagnosed only if the prolactin level is >800 mU/l on at least two occasions (there is overlap between normal and abnormal, and the level is also raised by stress, including attending hospital). Galactorrhoea occurs in <50% of those with hyperprolactinaemia, and <50% of those with galactorrhoea have an elevated prolactin level. If there is a normal menstrual cycle hyperprolactinaemia is unlikely to be of clinical significance.

Causes

Adenomas

These occur in the lateral wings of the anterior pituitary and are usually soft and discrete with a pseudocapsule of compressed tissue. If the Prl is >1000 mU/l, then imaging with CT or (ideally) MRI should be carried out; a microadenoma is <10 mm and a macroadenoma >10 mm. Serum levels correlate well with tumour size, a macroadenoma usually secreting at least 2500–3000 mU/l. If the Prl level is <2000–3000 mU/l with a tumour >10 mm, then pituitary stalk compression from a non-secreting macroadenoma or other tumour is possible (e.g. a craniopharyngioma). If the Prl level is >8000 mU/l, an adenoma is likely. If there is a macroadenoma, also check visual fields and arrange a short synacthen test. One-third of adenomas regress spontaneously and <5% of microadenomas become macroadenomas.

Secondary hyperprolactinaemia
Outside pregnancy and lactation, this may occur secondary to primary hypothyroidism, chronic renal failure, stalk compression, PCOS or drugs (phenothiazines, haloperidol, metoclopramide, cimetidine, methyldopa, antihistamines, morphine). The modern lower doses of oestrogen in the COC do not usually elevate prolactin. Around 10% of those with PCOS also have an elevated prolactin level, although the mechanism remains obscure.

Idiopathic hyperprolactinaemia
This may be due to microadenomas not picked up by MRI. Prl levels are usually <2500 mU/l. The condition should still be treated as there is a risk of reduced libido and (if there is amenorrhoea) osteoporosis. HRT should only be considered in those with treated microadenomas and given only under very close supervision.

Medical treatment of adenomas or idiopathic hyperprolactinaemia
All patients should have a T4, TSH and pituitary imaging before treatment.

Bromocriptine Start 1.25 mg nocte with food and increase over weeks to a maintenance level of around 5–7.5 mg/day in divided doses as directed by the Prl levels. The Prl level returns to normal (aim for 200–300 mU/L) in 90% of patients, with restoration of periods in 70%. Many are unable to tolerate side-effects, however, with nausea and vomiting occurring in 50%. There may also be postural hypotension. Treatment reduces the tumour size (and induces fibrosis), although the size often increases again after treatment is stopped.

Cabergoline If bromocriptine is not tolerated, use cabergoline 0.25 mg twice weekly (increasing to a maximum of 1 mg twice weekly) as the side-effect profile is better. Although there are no recognized teratogenic problems, there are only limited data on pregnancy safety (bromocriptine is thought to be safe in pregnancy, see below)

Surgical treatment
Transnasal trans-sphenoidal microsurgical excision is rarely used, and is reserved for those tumours resistant to medical therapy where there is suprasellar or frontal extension, or where stalk compression is suspected. The recurrence is 90% with macroadenomas and 40% with microadenomas. CSF rhinorrhoea occurs in 20%, transient diabetes insipidus is common and there are long-term hypopituitary problems in about 20%.

Pregnancy and lactation
In pregnancy, discontinue dopamine agonist treatment as soon as pregnancy is confirmed. The high levels of pregnancy-related prolactin renders prolactin

measurement of little value as a disease marker. There is a risk of tumour expansion in pregnancy, probably <5% with macroadenomas and <2% with microadenomas. In those known previously to have macroadenomas, arrange regular formal visual field testing. Those with microadenomas should probably simply be reviewed and advised to attend if there are headaches or visual-field symptoms. Breast-feeding is not contraindicated.

INFECTIONS

PELVIC INFLAMMATORY DISEASE (PID)

> The UK incidence is 1–2% per year amongst sexually active women, although this decreases with increasing age. It is associated with early age at first intercourse, is likely to occur at the time of menstruation and is less likely with COC and condom use. Infection ascends, possibly assisted by proteolytic enzymes and the motility of sperm or protozoa, to cause a primary infection. This may recur (either through reactivation or by repeated exposure) or may become chronic following secondary infection with endogenous organisms (usually polymicrobial). Infection may progress to pelvic abscess formation. Uterine instrumentation, especially at the time of TOP, also increases the risk of PID. The 'classical' picture of febrile illness, raised ESR and palpable adnexal swelling is seen in only 16% of those with laparoscopically proven PID.

If the diagnosis is based on:

- All three of
  - abdominal tenderness,
  - cervical excitation,
  - adnexal tenderness,
- and at least one of
  - temperature >38°C
  - WCC >10 × 10⁹/l,
  - ESR >15 mm/h,

then 70% will have salpingitis, 30% adhesions and 6% tubal occlusion at laparoscopy. Between 40% and 50% will be chlamydia positive (London-based study; Br J Obstet Gynaecol 1995:407).

There may also be:

- irregular PV bleeding (in 33%),
- vaginal discharge (in 50%),
- elevated CRP (80%).

The true incidence of PID is likely to be higher than cases identified using these criteria as a significant proportion of cases, particularly those with chlamydia, may have minimal symptoms or signs. Peak prevalence is at 15–25 years of age, raising important questions about whether this age group should be screened for subclinical infection (ideally using first-pass urine samples for PCR/LCR). Those undergoing induced abortion should be either screened for infection and treated before the procedure, or receive prophylactic antibiotics. It is also probable that those undergoing uterine instrumentation (including IUCD insertion, infertility laparoscopy and endometrial sampling), particularly in the 15–25 year age group, will benefit from screening.

Investigations

Take a history, carry out a clinical examination and check the WCC, ESR ± CRP. An endocervical swab (rotated to ensure that cells are taken) should be checked for chlamydia (or first-pass urine for LCR/PCR if available) and a further endocervical swab placed in Amies transport medium prior to culture for both *Neisseria gonorrhoeae* and anaerobes. Although the gold standard test for PID is laparoscopic evidence of tubal inflammation, laparoscopy is usually only carried out if there is a pelvic mass, failure to respond to treatment, or significant doubt about the diagnosis.

Laparoscopic findings are as follows:

- Mild: hyperaemia, exudate, oedema with freely mobile tubes.
- Moderate: gross exudate with adherent tubes.
- Severe: tubo-ovarian mass, pyosalpinx or abscess.

Although many primary and most secondary infections are polymicrobial, some infections may fit specific syndromes (Table 5.7).

TABLE 5.7 Infections associated with PID

Organism	Age of patient	Length of illness	Temperature	Features
Chlamydia trachomatis	Young	7 days to several months	Usually normal	Often minimal clinical features, but there may be intermenstrual bleeding or urinary symptoms. Dyspareunia is also common
Anaerobes	Older	<3 days	>38°C	Often second or third infection. Often unwell
Neisseria gonorrhoea	Young	<3 days	>38°C	Is rare in the UK. Unwell and very tender
Streptococci, coagulase-negative staphylococci and actinomycoses				Are rare

Treatment

Initial treatment is usually blind, as delay in treatment increases the risks of infertility. (See p. 189 for specific treatment after identification of the organism.)
The choice of oral or IV treatment depends on the patient's condition:

- If the patient is clinically well:
  — doxycycline 100 mg BD PO for 14–28 days (or azithromycin 1 g stat. PO, see p. 190), *plus*
  — metronidazole 200 mg TID PO for 14–28 days.
- If the patient is clinically unwell:
  — azithromycin 1 g stat. PO (or doxycycline 100 mg BD PO for 14–28 days), *plus*
  — *either* Cefuroxime 750 mg IV TID (or gentamicin IV see p. 104) and metronidazole 500 mg IV TID,
  — *or* co-amoxiclav 1.2 g IV TID.

Long-term prognosis

There is a seven- to tenfold increase in the risk of ectopic pregnancy. The incidence of tubal infertility increases with increasing numbers of infections and is >50% in those who have had three or more infections. Contact tracing of chlamydia-positive patients is important as treatment of partners reduces the risk of new and recurrent cases. Treatment of asymptomatic chlamydia-positive women also reduces the incidence of PID. One-third of patients will have a recurrence within 1 year.

VAGINAL DISCHARGE

> Physiological vaginal discharge changes throughout the reproductive life, increasing as the oestrogen level increases (e.g. at puberty, in pregnancy or with the COC).

History

Is the discharge itchy (candida) or offensive (foreign body, *Trichomonas vaginalis* or bacterial vaginosis)? Is there any pain or fever (PID if abdominal pain, HSV if vulval pain)? A sexual history should be obtained, and if there is a new sexual partner the possibility of a STD arises. If so, consider referral to a genitourinary medicine clinic for diagnosis, treatment and contact tracing.

Management

Perform a speculum examination to see whether the discharge is vaginal or cervical:

- If the history is one of pruritus vulvae, the patient is well and the discharge is white, prescribe antifungal preparations (swabs for culture are optional).

Treatment is with clotrimazole (e.g. Canesten) pessaries 200 mg nocte for 3 nights or a single 500 mg pessary stat. ±clotrimazole cream applied BD. Fluconazole (Diflucan) 150 mg/day PO stat is also effective, but may have systemic side-effects, and should not be used in pregnancy (see Candida Infection, p. 190).

- If there is a creamy yellow discharge with an offensive smell, treat with metronidazole 200 mg TID PO for 7 days or with 2% clindamycin cream 5 g applicator nocte PV for 7 nights (see Bacterial Vaginosis below and *Trichomonas vaginalis*, p. 193).

- If there is no response to the above, or there are concerns about STDs, or there is an endocervical discharge, take swabs:
  — endocervical (Amies transport medium) for *N. gonorrhoea*;
  — high vaginal (Amies transport medium) for routine culture;
  — endocervical for *Chlamydia trachomatis* (or first-pass urine for PCR/LCR if available) and treat individual infections as outlined below;
  — if you have the experience, examination of a fresh wet smear may demonstrate *Trichomonas vaginalis*.

- If there has been no response to the above measures and there are no identifiable organisms, it is worth formally calling a halt to investigations and reviewing the original history. Discussion about the changing nature of a physiological discharge and reassurance about the absence of infection is often reassuring.

Treating a cervical ectropion to cure vaginal discharge is frequently unrewarding. Topical or systemic oestrogen treatment for recurrent vaginal infections may be of help in atrophic vaginitis (e.g. postmenopausally, those on depot progestogens).

SPECIFIC PELVIC INFECTIONS AND SEXUALLY TRANSMITTED DISEASES

With the possible exception of PID, this is best managed in an STD clinic with facilities for counselling, contact tracing and on-site Gram stain and microscopy.

Actinomycoses
This is a Gram-negative bacterium which only rarely causes salpingitis (often unilateral, more often on the right), chronic tubo-ovarian abscesses and fistulae. It may occur secondary to appendicitis or with IUCD use. It is not sexually transmitted. Treat with high-dose oral or parenteral penicillin.

Bacterial vaginosis
This occurs when lactobacilli are replaced by anaerobes, particularly bacteroides species. *Gardnerella vaginalis* probably has a small role. Bacterial vaginosis is not sexually transmitted and many women are

asymptomatic. The pH increases to ≈5.5 and bacterial metabolites produce volatile amines with a 'fishy' odour. The discharge is green or grey, thin and offensive. On wet microscopy there are epithelial cells surrounded by bacteria ('clue' cells). Treat with metronidazole 2 g stat. PO (or 200 mg BD for 7 days if recurrent), or with clindamycin cream 2% (5 g applicator nocte for 7 nights). If pregnant, ampicillin 500 mg PO QID may be a more appropriate oral treatment. There is no benefit in treating the partner or in using condoms.

Bacteroides spp.

These are commensals but may cause a vaginal discharge (see Bacterial Vaginosis, above) or complicate pre-existing PID (leading to chronic infection). They are not sexually transmitted. Treat with metronidazole 200 mg TID 7 days or with clindamycin cream 2% (5 g applicator nocte for 7 nights).

Candida or thrush (*Candida albicans*)

This is not sexually transmitted. It presents with a whitish discharge and pruritus. The vulva and vagina may be fissured and painful. It occurs more commonly in the sexually active, the pregnant and the immunocompromised. The COC probably makes no difference. Microscopy reveals yeasts and pseudohyphae and a high vaginal swab may be cultured on Sabouraud's medium. Treatment is with clotrimazole (e.g. Canesten) pessaries 200 mg nocte for 3 nights or a single 500 mg pessary stat. ±clotrimazole cream applied BD. Fluconazole (Diflucan) 150 mg/day PO stat. is also effective, but may have systemic side-effects, and should not be used in pregnancy. If proven infection is recurrent there is no benefit from treating the partner. Prophylactic treatment, however, may be of benefit. (For example, if the patient's symptoms are particularly troublesome premenstrually, insert a single pessary midcycle). Alternatively, a weekly pessary may be used; 100, 200 or 500 mg, depending on which dose controls the symptoms. Natural yoghurt on a tampon nocte for 3 nights, acetic acid jelly (e.g. Aci-Jel), wiping the anus front to back, and cotton underwear may also be of help.

Chlamydia (*Chlamydia trachomatis* serovars D–K)

This is the commonest bacterial sexually transmitted infection in the UK (0.5–15% depending on sample selected), and is a much commoner cause of infection than the gonococcus. In the female it is often asymptomatic, but may cause PID, bartholinitis, spontaneous abortion, premature labour, neonatal conjunctivitis (5–14 days postnatally) and neonatal pneumonia. PID with associated perihepatitis is known as the Fitz–Hugh–Curtis syndrome. Reiter syndrome (arthritis, mucosal ulceration, conjunctival symptoms) is very rare in women. In the male *C. trachomatis* infection may cause urethral discharge, dysuria, epididymo-orchitis and Reiter syndrome. Diagnosis in the female is by endocervical swabs, urethral swabs or first-void urine sent in a specific transport medium for LCR or PCR.

Uncomplicated infection my be treated with azithromycin (Zithromax) 1 g (four 250 mg capsules) stat. PO (great compliance benefit), or doxycycline 200 mg stat. PO then 100 mg/day for 7 days, or erythromycin 500 mg BD for 7 days (all equally effective assuming there are no compliance problems). There is no evidence that azithromycin is adequate for chlamydial salpingitis, but it is likely that it provides adequate cover. Increased doses plus the addition of metronidazole are employed for complicated infection (see PID, p. 186). Test of cure is not essential (swabs may remain positive for up to 4 weeks despite adequate treatment), but contact tracing is important and individuals should avoid unprotected intercourse for 2 weeks.

Genital warts

These are usually caused by HPV 6 and 11, though occasionally 16 and 18. Most patients with genital HPV have no visible warts but the virus can be transmitted to sexual partners who may then develop visible lesions. Of those with warts, 25% have other demonstrable STDs. Podophyllin paint can be applied weekly to the non-pregnant patient by medical staff, with advice to wash the solution off 6 hours later. Self-treatment is also available with podophyllotoxin solution (e.g. Condyline or Warticon). This is applied BD for 3 days, repeating on a weekly cycle for four weeks. For patients with multiple, large warts only a few should be treated at a time, as severe discomfort has been reported. Warts may be treated with cryotherapy using liquid nitrogen, or be lasered or diathermized under GA. Immune stimulators (e.g. Imiquimod, 3M Healthcare) are occasionally considered for recalcitrant warts; treatment is expensive and not of definite proven value. Annual cervical screening is not required, but those with visible cervical warts or abnormal cytology should be colposcoped.

Gonorrhoea (*Neisseria gonorrhoea*)

The incubation period is 2–5 days for men. The vast majority of women are asymptomatic, but infection may cause PID (often at time of menstruation), urethritis, polyarthralgia, miscarriage, premature labour and neonatal ophthalmia (2–7 days postnatally). Most men have symptoms of urethritis and discharge. Swabs should be taken from the urethra and cervix and placed in Amies transport medium. A Gram stain of an endocervical swab shows Gram-negative intracellular diplococci in only 50%, so that definitive diagnosis is by culture on NYC medium. Treatment is with ampicillin 2–4 g PO stat. together with probenecid 1 g PO stat. Ciprofloxacin (Ciproxin) 250 mg PO stat. is used in penicillin allergy and for infections acquired in regions where resistance is common (take advice from the microbiology department).

Herpes (herpes simplex virus)

This infection classically occurs secondary to the sexually transmitted type II virus, but infection with type I from coldsores is increasingly common. The incubation is 2–14 days, with itch and dysuria being prominent early symptoms. The vulva becomes ulcerated and exquisitely painful and, in the first attack (which may last 3–4 weeks), there may be systemic flu-like symptoms ±secondary bacterial infection. Autoinnoculation to fingers and eyes can occur and there may be a sacral radiculopathy giving a self-limiting paraesthesia to the buttocks and thighs. Only very rarely is there an associated meningitis or encephalitis. Strong oral or IM analgesia and advice to micturate while in the bath may be of help (lignocaine gel is painful to apply and may lead to hypersensitivity reactions). Aciclovir 200 mg PO 5-hourly shortens the duration of symptoms and lessens infectivity (famciclovir and valiciclovir are alternatives). Recurrent infections are shorter (lasting 5–10 days) and usually less severe. Recurrence of infection in the first year is 95% in type II and 5% in type I infections. Aciclovir cream should be used at the start of subsequent infections. Prophylactic oral aciclovir 400 mg PO BD should be reserved for those with frequent incapacitating infections (e.g. >10/year) and should be continued for at least 12 months. There is no necessity for annual cervical cytology. (See Infection in Pregnancy, p. 134).

HIV infection
(See page 136).

Lymphogranuloma venereum (tropical; *Chlamydia trachomatis* serovars L1–L3)
This is a chronic disease beginning with primary ulceration, followed 4 days to 4 months later by secondary lymphoedema and regional lymphadenitis. Treat with doxycycline 100 mg/day PO for 14 days.

Streptococci or coagulase-negative staphylococci
These may complicate pre-existing PID. Treat with ampicillin 500 mg PO QID for 7 days and metronidazole 400 mg TID for 7 days. (See Pregnancy p. 137).

Syphilis (*Treponema pallidum*)
A primary chancre (raised, round, indurated usually painless ulcer) resolves in 3–8 weeks and may be followed by secondary fever, headaches, bone and joint pain, generalized rash, condylomata lata and generalized painless lymphadenopathy. Following the latent phase there may be tertiary gummas or quaternary neurological and cardiovascular disease. Congenital syphilis may lead to IUD or midtrimester loss. Survivors may be premature, have IUGR, Hutchinson's triad and nasal discharge. The diagnosis is made serologically, with most laboratories using the VDRL, TPHA and FTA tests. Many laboratories now screen with an antitreponemal IgG ELISA which is highly sensitive but does give false-positive results. True positive results are confirmed by the more traditional tests. Treatment is with procaine penicillin 900 mg/day IM for 10–21 days depending on the stage of the disease.

Trichomonas vaginalis

This is usually sexually transmitted. There is a foul-smelling, purulent vaginal discharge with accompanying symptoms of dysuria and vulval soreness. Diagnosis is by identification on a wet film. Treat with metronidazole as for bacterial vaginosis.

INFERTILITY

Subfertility is an involuntary failure to conceive within 12 months of commencing unprotected intercourse, and may be primary or secondary. The incidence of primary infertility is at least 12% of couples (for causes see Table 5.8). A coital history is essential. *Both partners must be investigated.*

CAUSES

The causes of infertility are given in Table 5.8. Note that the sum of the causes in the table is >100% as there may be more than one factor. Many couples have subfertility with specific partners. When there is a mild defect in one there is an increased likelihood of finding a mild defect in the other as well.

TABLE 5.8 Causes of infertility

Female cause	Unknown cause	Male cause
15% Tubal problem	25% Idiopathic	40%
20% Anovulation	5% Sexual problem	
10% Other		

INVESTIGATION

Female factor infertility

History

As well as a general medical, surgical and family history, take a menstrual history and ask about galactorrhoea and hirsutism. Confirm that the woman is taking folic acid 0.4 mg/day to reduce the incidence of neural tube defects (see p. 14). Both men and women should give up smoking. Women should not drink more than 2–4 units of alcohol per week, and men should limit their drinking.

Examination

Check the BMI (diet if >30). Carry out a general medical examination, looking particularly for thyroid swelling, galactorrhoea and hirsutism. Also, carry out a pelvic examination and check a cervical smear if appropriate.

Investigations

Confirm ovulation In a menstruating woman, the diagnosis is based on a midluteal (i.e. 1 week *before the next period*) serum progesterone >30 nmol/l, or a urine pregnandiol >0.5 mmol/ml (samples can be collected weekly). If there is no ovulation in a young woman with no history to suggest PID or endometriosis, it *may* be worth undertaking ovulation induction for 4 months (months) prior to confirming tubal patency (providing the semen analysis of her partner is normal). If there is anovulation, check early follicular Prl (see p. 184), LH, FSH, T$_4$, TSH and testosterone (see PCOS, p. 182).

Rubella antibodies Check and, if negative, immunize and advise contraception for 3 months before rechecking serology.
? 1 mo

Confirmation of tubal patency This may be by laparoscopy and dye insufflation of the fallopian tubes or by hysterosalpingogram. *The patient must not be pregnant*. Laparoscopy allows exclusion of PID and endometriosis, and avascular peritubal adhesions may be divided (the treatment of vascular adhesions gives poor results). Salpingostomy for tubal blockage carries conception rates little more than ≈20% and IVF may be more appropriate. Tubal surgery should probably be carried out in a specialist centre.

Male factor infertility

History
This should include alcohol, smoking, sexual development, surgery (particularly maldescent, hernias, varicocele or prostate), urinary problems (? structural abnormality), orchitis (including mumps), recent systemic infections (may temporarily lower the sperm count) and occupation (exposure to toxins). Erectile function should also be discussed (e.g. IDDM, MS, drugs).

Examination ·
Carry out a general medical examination, looking particularly at secondary sexual characteristics. In the urogenital examination look for inguinal scars and check the urethral orifice. Assess the site and size of the testis, confirm the presence of the vas and exclude varicocele or epididymal cysts. Infertile men have an increased risk of testicular cancer.

Investigations
Semen analysis varies widely from ejaculate to ejaculate, and two results should be sought at least 1 month apart. Samples should be kept warm in the patient's pocket and brought to the laboratory ASAP (<1–2 hours).
A 'normal' semen analysis is not proof of ability to fertilize an ovum.

WHO criteria for 'normal' semen analysis			
Volume:	> 2 ml	Morphology:	>40% normal
pH:	7–8	Alive:	>50%
Concentration:	>20 × 10⁶/ml	WCC:	<1 × 10⁶
Motility:	>50% forward	Antisperm antibodies	
	>25% with rapid linear progress	(MAR test):	negative

If the semen analysis is abnormal check LH, FSH, Prl, testosterone and antisperm antibodies. Advise wearing loose-fitting underwear and recheck in 12 weeks. Additional investigations include in vitro tests of sperm–mucus interaction. The postcoital test is not recommended in the routine investigation of infertility, but may be of value if there are real doubts about sexual function. Intrauterine insemination is only of value when combined with superovulation, but the increase in the pregnancy rate remains low.

Azoospermia If the FSH is increased there is testicular failure. Check chromosomes. If the FSH is normal there is an obstruction. Is the vas present? (It is absent in cystic fibrosis.) If present, consider scrotal exploration and microsurgical repair. Testicular biopsy will allow recovery of sufficient spermatozoa for ICSI in >50% of men, even those with elevated FSH.

Oligospermia, teratospermia (abnormal morphology) or asthenospermia (poor motility) Specific causes are rare. Review the history of alcohol, drugs, etc. If a varicocele is present, consider referral to radiologists for embolization, as varicocele treatment improves sperm quality and probably pregnancy rates in oligospermia.

Specific endocrine causes Hyperprolactinaemia usually causes loss of libido (see p. 184). Hypogonadotrophic hypogonadism (low LH, FSH and testosterone) responds well to a GnRH pump or LH + FSH by injection.

Remember
Many couples with male factor infertility will conceive naturally. In the absence of a specific aetiology, the only treatments are donor insemination or IVF (with or without microsurgical fertilization, depending on the severity of the problem).

Both partners

If investigations of both the man and the woman are normal, the couple should be reviewed. If they are young and have been trying for a relatively short time (e.g. 2 years), it is appropriate to reassure them and adopt a 'wait and see policy' (60–70% of couples will conceive spontaneously in the following 2 years). In unexplained infertility assisted reproduction may be appropriate after 3–4 years, although perhaps earlier if age is a major factor. Ovarian stimulation with intrauterine insemination may also be of benefit in this group. Treatment with clomiphene is not warranted in unexplained ovulatory infertility.

OVULATION INDUCTION

In a menstruating woman, the diagnosis of ovulation is based on a midluteal (i.e. 1 week *before the next period*) serum progesterone >30 nmol/l or a urine pregnandiol >0.5 mmol/ml. If the patient has amenorrhoea, exclude pregnancy and give Provera 5 mg TID for 5 days (or gestodene 100 mg IM stat.). If there is a withdrawal bleed use antioestrogens. If there is no bleed, gonadotrophin injections or pulsatile GnRH may be indicated.

Antioestrogens These compete with natural oestrogens by blocking receptors in the pituitary, leading to increased FSH levels. Clomiphene (Clomid) is the initial drug of choice, beginning at 50 mg/day PO from days 3–7 of the cycle. The incidence of multiple pregnancy is ≈10%. Other side-effects are rare, but include visual disturbances (an indication for withdrawal), hot flushes, breast tenderness, abdominal discomfort and rashes (there have been recent concerns about an increase in the risk of ovarian cancer when clomiphene is used for more than 12 cycles, but this association remains unproven). Ovarian hyperstimulation is rare, and usually resolves spontaneously. Check a 21 day progesterone level or track weekly urine samples to look for evidence of ovulation.

If there is a spontaneous bleed beginning around days 28–35 the clomiphene should be restarted again for 5 days, again beginning on day 3. If there has been no bleed by day 42, exclude pregnancy and give Provera 10 mg PO BD for 5 days. A withdrawal bleed should be expected within a few days of stopping Provera, and Clomiphene again restarted as above. If there has been no ovulation after 2 cycles on 50 mg/day it is reasonable to increase the dose to 100 mg/day PO over the same 5 days for 2 months, then 150 mg for a further 2 months to a maximum 200 mg/day. If there is no ovulation and the testosterone level has been elevated, dexamethasone 0.5 mg/day may be given in the follicular phase of the cycle up to the time of ovulation. Failure of oral treatment suggests the need for gonadotrophin therapy. Laparoscopic ovarian drilling with either diathermy or laser is an effective treatment for anovulation in women with clomiphene resistant PCOS.

Gonadotrophin therapy This should only be carried out with very careful monitoring. Low-dose gonadotrophin injections may be started within a few days of a bleed in a menstruating woman or at any time in amenorrhoea. Injections are given daily and follicle stimulation monitored with USS and serum oestradiol. When one follicle is >16 mm, hCG is given and the couple advised to have intercourse. Luteal support with hCG is not required (and increases the risk of multiple pregnancy and ovarian hyperstimulation syndrome). If initial gonadotrophins are normal or elevated, it may be useful to suppress the HPO axis before treatment with an IM or intranasal GnRH analogue. The multiple pregnancy rate is 20–30% and there is a significant risk of hyperstimulation. Many of these women have PCOS and there is a high spontaneous abortion rate (≈30%). Purified or recombinant FSH have advantages over older hMG preparations.

Pulsatile GnRH analogue This is a pulsatile SC (or IV) infusion of GnRH by a miniaturized automatic infusion system. Treatment is monitored using ultrasound measurement of follicular development. After ovulation, the pulsatile infusion may be discontinued and luteal support provided. This is a very effective treatment in hypogonadotrophic hypogonadism and usually results in the development of a single follicle.

Hyperstimulation

Ovarian hyperstimulation syndrome is an iatrogenic complication of ovulation induction, usually associated with gonadotrophin use. It is reported to occur in 0.6–14% of IVF cycles and is characterized by increased vascular permeability, which can lead to fluid in the serous cavities (usually ascites, occasionally pleural and only rarely a pericardial effusion). It tends to be more prolonged and severe if pregnancy occurs, but is nonetheless self-limiting. Fatalities occur, albeit rarely.

Classification of ovarian hyperstimulation syndrome

Mild
- Abdominal bloating, mild pain
- Ovarian size usually <8 cm

Moderate
- Increased pain, nausea, diarrhoea
- Ovarian size usually 8–12 cm with ascites

Severe
- Clinical ascites, haemoconcentration (Hct >45%, WBC >15 000/ml)
- Oliguria with normal creatinine
- Liver dysfunction
- Ovarian size usually <12 cm

Critical
- Tense ascites (Hct >55%, WBC >25 000/ml)
- Renal failure
- Thromboembolic phenomena

Treatment

- Liaise with the assisted conception unit if possible.
- Check U&E, FBC (increased haematocrit), LFTs, albumin and clotting. Arrange a USS of the ovaries; look also for ascites.

- Analgesia with paracetamol or with opiates if required.
- Push oral fluids to avoid haemoconcentration. Aim to maintain blood volume and urine output, if necessary using IV crystalloid (normal saline). If haemoconcentration is severe (>44%) consider colloid±CVP monitoring.
- Prevent thromboses with support stockings and heparin 5000 U SC BD.
- Abdominal paracentesis is practised aggressively by some and gives good symptomatic relief, but it will accentuate the protein loss. It will relieve respiratory compromise and is occasionally useful if oliguria is secondary to pressure of tense ascites on the renal veins.
- The most serious cases may also require drainage of effusions and a dopamine infusion to maintain renal function.
- Surgery should only be undertaken for a ruptured cyst or haemorrhage and by a very experienced operator. TOP may very rarely be required.

ASSISTED REPRODUCTION

Entry guidelines to assisted reproduction units vary, but an example would be: a clear positive recommendation from the GP in a couple with no more than one previous child in a continuing heterosexual relationship of at least 2 years' duration. The woman should be <40 years old and in good health. (There is no legal requirement for any of these factors.) The couple should be aware of the immense emotional strain involved. The success rate (i.e. 'take home baby rate' for GIFT and IVF is ≈20%). The incidence of spontaneous abortion is increased, as are the risks of multiple pregnancy (≈25%), antenatal bleeds, PIH (? because of the older population), breech presentation, preterm labour (may be iatrogenic) and SFD neonates. There is no increase in the incidence of congenital abnormality.

IVF

This may be indicated for tubal disease, unexplained infertility, endometriosis, male factor infertility, failed donor insemination or cervical hostility. Donor oocytes may be used with failed ovaries (e.g. Turner syndrome, premature menopause). 'Superovulation' is used for oocyte harvest. HPO down-regulation is achieved initially with GnRH analogues (IM or intranasally) and is followed by hMG or FSH in much larger doses than is used for ovulation induction: 5000 U Profasi is given when there are >3 follicles >16 mm in diameter. Oocyte retrieval 32–34 hours later is usually carried out transvaginally under systemic sedation using ultrasound-guided needle aspiration, although laparoscopy may be used. Approximately 10% of cycles are abandoned before oocyte harvest, usually in older patients or in those with endometriosis, because of poor ovarian response. Cycles may also be cancelled because of hyperstimulation.

Spermatozoa are prepared and added to the oocyte. At 48 hours after oocyte recovery, a fine plastic cannula is used to place a maximum of three (ideally ≤2) embryos 1 cm from the uterine fundus. 'Surplus' embryos can be cryopreserved and replaced 2 days after ovulation in a natural cycle. Luteal support is usually given in IVF or embryo transfer cycles.

GIFT

This is suitable for all those mentioned under IVF except for those with blocked or absent fallopian tubes. Oocytes are collected laparoscopically, mixed with sperm and transferred to the fimbrial end of the fallopian tube. This technique does not involve such advanced embryological back-up and may be carried out in smaller centres.

ICSI (intracytoplasmic sperm injection)

This involves the in vitro injection of a sperm into an oocyte. The advantages are that any type of sperm (sperm head, immotile sperm, defective sperm) can be injected and that both capacitation and acrosome reaction are unnecessary for fertilization. Sperm can be harvested from the epididymis or testis and very small numbers of sperm have been used successfully. Although this technique requires advanced embryological back-up, it is revolutionizing the treatment of severe male factor infertility. It is associated with a very small risk of sex chromosome abnormalities and the long-term risks (e.g. infertility in male offspring) are uncertain.

MENOPAUSE

> The average age at onset of the menopause in the UK is 51 years and is unaffected by parity, age at menarche, or use of the COC (it occurs 6–18 months earlier in smokers). Eight per cent reach the menopause before the age of 40 years (see Premature Ovarian Failure, p. 209). Anovulatory cycles and luteal inadequacy are more common after 40 years of age and may lead to DUB ± endometrial hyperplasia.

Clinical features

Approximately 30% of women are not significantly troubled by flushing or sweating, while these vasomotor symptoms are mild or moderate in ≥30% and severe in the remaining ≥30%. Seventy-five per cent experience flushing or sweating for more than 1 year and 25% for more than 5 years, sometimes much more. Vasomotor symptoms can last from 1 minute to 1 hour and be associated with panic attacks, fatigue and insomnia. Decreased genital blood supply and genital atrophy occur, with loss of hair, elasticity and muscle tone. Vaginal moisture and lubrication are reduced. Anxiety, irritability and depression may be more common after the menopause and libido may decrease.

Longer term problems may arise, with loss of skin thickness and loss of the cardioprotective effect of oestrogens. There is rapid bone loss for a few years after the menopause and after cessation of HRT. Osteoporosis may result. Men have 20% more bone at peak skeletal maturity and fractures are eight times commoner (age for age) than in men. Alzheimer's disease is commoner in women and may be reduced by postmenopausal oestrogen therapy.

Diagnosis

𝔇𝑫

The menopause may be confused with PMS, depression, thyroid dysfunction, pregnancy and, rarely, phaeochromocytoma or carcinoid syndrome. Prolactinoma should be excluded, especially in younger women. Vasomotor symptoms may be caused by calcium antagonists and by depressive therapy, especially tricyclics.

Postmenopausally the FSH should be >30 u/l, but perimenopausally the level may be normal. A midcycle peak of FSH and an early-cycle low oestradiol may cause confusion in a premenopausal woman. If there is diagnostic doubt, especially over 45 years of age, a therapeutic trial of HRT may be undertaken. Absence of a satisfactory response suggests that symptoms may not be genuinely menopausal.

Hormone replacement therapy

HRT improves vasomotor flushes and sweats, mood problems and vaginal dryness in most patients. There is also a major reduction in ischaemic heart disease long term (RR = 0.48), with the possible exception of women with well-advanced heart disease at the onset of HRT. The incidence of cerebrovascular disease is neither increased or decreased. Osteoporotic fractures may be reduced by 50%.

For those between the ages of 50 and 70 years, the incidence of breast carcinoma is increased from a baseline of 45:1000 to 47:1000 after 5 years, to 51:1000 after 10 years and 57:1000 after 15 years (Lancet 1997;350:1047). There is no increased risk in those who stopped taking HRT more than 5 years previously. It may be that breast cancer diagnosed while on HRT is 20% more curable, and HRT containing oestrogen is therefore probably relatively safe for 10 years after the age of 50.

Unopposed therapy (i.e. oestrogen only) increases the incidence of endometrial cancer fourfold, and should be used only for those who have had a hysterectomy. The incidence is reduced to a RR of less than 1 with opposed therapy (i.e. with the addition of progesterone for 12 days per cycle). The levonorgestrel releasing intrauterine system (Mirena) protects the endometrium effectively when used in conjunction with oestrogen HRT in postmenopausal women.

There is also an increased risk of venous thromboembolic disease in the first year of treatment (Br Med J 1997;314:796), with a RR of 4.6 in the first 6 months and 3.0 in the second 6 months (baseline risk 1.3:1000 per year).

There is apparently no increased risk in those taking it beyond 1 year. Routine pretreatment screening for thrombophilia is not recommended, but should be carried out in those with a personal or family history of venous thromboembolic disease (RCOG Guideline No. 19, 1999).

Use of oestrogen-containing HRT is widely considered to be contraindicated following breast carcinoma (including intraduct carcinoma). A number of publications report no ill effects, but the power of their statistics may be insufficient. HRT is also avoided following advanced endometrial carcinoma, but combined HRT has been shown to be safe in early disease (Intl J Gynaecol Cancer 1994;4:217).

Fluid retention, breast pain, perceived weight gain (often more related to calorie intake than HRT) and withdrawal bleeds are common reasons for discontinuing HRT. Unexplained vaginal bleeding and the possibility of pregnancy are contraindications.

Oral preparations The oral route may have a more beneficial effect than parenteral therapy on lipid profiles, leading to increased HDL and decreased LDL. It is possibly less beneficial to coagulation factors in view of the first-pass liver effect.

Cyclical preparations are used perimenopausally, while cyclical or continuous combined therapy are options postmenopausally (more than 2 years from the last period). Continuous combined therapy is more convenient in the ≥70% who do not suffer unscheduled bleeding, but erratic bleeing beyond the first 6 months of treatment in those who do suffer unscheduled bleeding warrants further investigation. Tibolone (Livial) is a synthetic steroid with weak oestrogenic, progestogenic and androgenic effects which may also be started 2 years after periods have ceased. Raloxifene (Evista 60 mg/day), a selective oestrogen-receptor modulator, has oestrogenic effects on bone and lipid metabolism but has a minimal effect on uterine or breast tissues (N Engl J Med 1997:1641). It is ineffective for controlling perimenopausal symptoms (and may cause flushings in a small proportion of women).

Unopposed progestogens (norethisterone 5–10 mg/day, or medroxyprogesterone acetate 10–20 mg/day) may be employed following breast cancer, endometrial cancer, venous thromboembolic disease and severe endometriosis, giving vasomotor symptom control in about 60% of subjects. Only norethisterone protects the skeleton.

Transdermal patches These are available with unopposed oestrogen, cyclical oestrogen and continuous oestrogen–progestogen. The first-pass liver effect is avoided and they have less effect on lipid metabolism and hepatic coagulation factors. Some studies claim a favourable effect on other cardiovascular protective mechanisms. Five per cent or more of subjects suffer skin reactions, ranging from hyperaemia to blisters, especially with alcohol-based adhesive patches.

Percutaneous gels A measured dose of oestradiol is rubbed through the skin, avoiding the prolonged skin contact of patches.

Subcutaneous implants Oestradiol may be implanted in subcutaneous fat, usually lower abdominally, administering 25–50 mg at intervals of no less than 5–6 months. The oestradiol level does not always fall away to baseline before symptoms recur, and there is a danger of 'tachyphylaxis' with ever-increasing oestradiol levels and persistent symptoms if strict control of dose is not observed. Monitor preimplant oestradiol levels aiming for <300–600 pmol/l. Testosterone implants (100 mg) may be used to increase energy and libido. This does not work for all women, but some find it effective.

Vaginal preparations Tablets of oestradiol 0.025 mg, low-dose oestradiol releasing silastic ring pessaries and oestriol vaginal pessaries or vaginal cream may be employed for atrophic vaginitis or trigonitis.

MENORRHAGIA AND DYSMENORRHOEA

The menstrual cycle is most regular between 20 and 40 years of age, with a tendency towards a longer cycle after menarche and a shorter one before the menopause. The mean menstrual blood loss in the healthy European population is ≈40 ml with 70% lost in the first 48 hours. Only 10% lose more than 80 ml (60% of these become anaemic). The actual blood loss correlates poorly with symptoms.

Causes of menorrhagia

No identifiable pelvic pathology This is the situation in the majority of cases, i.e. dysfunctional uterine bleeding (DUB). The cycles may be:

- Anovulatory (10%): this may occur in early adolescence, premenopausally or with PCOS. The cycles are generally irregular and there may be a risk of cystic glandular hyperplasia.
- Ovulatory (90%): this is usually idiopathic or may be due to an inadequate luteal phase following poor luteal follicular development.

Identifiable pathology

- Fibroids: 50% of those with menstrual loss >200 ml have fibroids.
- Foreign body: e.g. non-progestogen secreting IUCD.
- The role of PID and polyps is unclear.

Medical problems Particularly hypothyroidism, Cushing's syndrome, bleeding disorders (e.g. with von Willebrand's disease or thrombocytopenia, and usually not in those on warfarin, heparin or with coagulation disorders). Medical problems are very rare causes of menorrhagia.

Classification of dysmenorrhoea
This may be:

- Primary (i.e. idiopathic): this often occurs in the teenage years and may be related to elevated PGF-2α levels. Prescribing the COC is frequently of benefit.
- Secondary: to fibroids, the IUCD, PID, endometriosis or adenomyosis.

Investigations

These should include a history (including drugs and thyroid symptoms) and clinical examination. It is also important to assess the effects on lifestyle and general well-being. Check a FBC (TFTs only if symptomatic; no other endocrine tests are necessary). Endometrial assessment (see p. 205) should be undertaken in those >40 years if the periods are irregular or if there has been a recent change in the menses. The risk of endometrial malignancy in women <40 years old is between 1:10000 and 1:100000, rising to approximately 1:100 premenopausally.

Medical treatment

PG synthesis inhibitors For example, mefanamic acid (Ponstan) 500 mg TID taken at the time of bleeding reduces the mean blood loss by 20–40% in those with menorrhagia. It is also useful for dysmenorrhea. *Side-effects*: 50% have GI problems and 20% experience dizziness or headaches.

Antifibrinolytics For example, tranxenamic acid (Cyclokapron) 1 g BD to QID during the time of bleeding reduces mean blood loss by 50% in those with DUB or IUCD related menorrhagia. *Side-effects*: nausea, vomiting, tinnitus, rash and abdominal cramps. *Contraindications*: a history of thromboembolic disease.

Progestogens For example, medroxyprogesterone acetate (Provera) 5 mg TID on days 5–24 reduces blood loss in DUB (even if the cycles are regular). It is likely that 5 mg TID on days 16–24 has no benefit in those with regular cycles. *Side-effects*: oedema, bloating and weight gain, as well as androgenic problems. Use additional contraception.

COCs These are useful, particularly in younger, non-smoking patients, reducing blood loss by ≈50%. They may also be used continuously, e.g. two or three packets may be run together making periods less frequent.

Levonorgestrel impregnated IUCD (Mirena) This acts locally within the uterus to prevent proliferation of the endometrium, and reduces menstrual loss by an average of 90% after 3 months' treatment. Initial worsening of symptoms is common and intermenstrual bleeding occurs frequently, but these problems often settle 5 or 6 months after insertion. Twenty per cent of women experience complete amenorrhoea. Side-effects of lower abdominal discomfort (≈10%), skin problems (≈5%), and mastalgia (≈4%) have been reported, but these figures have not been compared to a control group. There is no change in weight or blood pressure. Mirena has a contraceptive licence for 3 years in the UK, but this may be increased to 5 years in the near future (in line with other European countries); there is good evidence that it remains effective in menstrual dysfunction for up to 7 or 8 years. (Br J Obstet Gynaecol 1998:592).

Danazol (Danol) This is of no use if taken cyclically. Start with 200 mg/day on a continuous basis. It reduces blood loss, but it may be necessary to increase to 200 mg BD or TID if amenorrhoea is required. *Side-effects*: weight gain, acne, hirsutism, cramps, headaches and breast atrophy (if severe). Use additional contraception.

GnRH analogues These are expensive and lead to both flushings and hypo-oestrogenic side-effects, particularly osteoporosis. (See p. 179.)

Surgical treatment

Abdominal and vaginal hysterectomy See page 221.

Alternatives There are a number of alternatives to traditional hysterectomy available using minimal access techniques. The round and broad ligaments may be divided laparoscopically, allowing removal of the ovaries by vaginal hysterectomy (laparoscopically assisted vaginal hysterectomy). Additionally, the uterine arteries may be taken. The entire hysterectomy may be performed laparoscopically, with removal of the specimen piecemeal through either the posterior fornix or one of the lateral ports.

Endometrial ablation All techniques are reported to have good short-term results with ≈80% satisfied at 1 year, although amenorrhoea occurs in only 20–30%. There are a number of possible operations, and all are only suitable for those who have completed their families. The operation is not in itself a contraceptive and pregnancy following the operation carries a high complication rate. Effective contraception is therefore essential and sterilization is ideal. The incidence of complications is about 12% particularly of haemorrhage, infection, perforation and damage to surrounding structures. With the first two techniques there is an additional risk of fluid overload which may occur if the fluid deficit is more than ≈1500–2000 ml. It presents with increased BP, decreased Na, neurological symptoms and ARDS. In those planning subsequent HRT at any stage, combined preparations should be used. Endometrial preparation for laser or TCRE is required 4–6 weeks preoperatively with danazol 200 mg TID or one of the GnRH analogues (see p. 179).

- *TCRE (transcervical endometrial resection).* Direct vision is used to ablate the endometrium using cutting diathermy. It is also possible to carry out additional surgery, including resection of submucous fibroids. The technique is relatively difficult to learn. Rollerball diathermy is an alternative.
- *The laser (Nd-YAG).* This can be used to ablate the endometrium under endoscopic vision. The technique is also relatively difficult to learn.
- *Ablation with a heated intrauterine water-filled balloon* (Thermachoice).

- *Ablation using a multi-electrode balloon* (Vesta DUB Treatment system).
- *MEA (microwave endometrial ablation).*
- *RAFEA (radiofrequency endometrial ablation).*

POSTMENOPAUSAL BLEEDING

Postmenopausal bleeding is defined as bleeding from the genital tract, either 6 months or 1 year following cessation of the menses. Around 10% of women with PMB have a primary or secondary malignancy, most commonly endometrial cancer (80%), cervical cancer or an ovarian tumour. Approximately 90%, therefore, have a benign cause, usually genital tract atrophy. Polyps are found in 5–9%, endometrial hyperplasia in up to 10% and extragenital pathology in 4%.

Investigations

Whether hysteroscopy or ultrasound, combined with endometrial sampling, is used depends on patient risk factors and local facilities. Pathology can be missed by any of these methods.

Dilatation and curettage Used alone this will miss 15% of endometrial cancers.

Hysteroscopy This will miss significant pathology in only 3% of cases.

Endometrial biopsy The pipelle and the vabra aspirator are the most commonly used tools in the UK. They are both 3 mm diameter, the pipelle being a thin plastic tube and the vabra a stainless-steel device used with an electrical suction pump. The pipelle is the most convenient, best tolerated and least expensive, but samples only around 4% of the endometrial surface and has a sensitivity of 67–97% (J Reprod Med 1995;40:553). The vabra samples around 40% of the endometrial surface but is more painful and more expensive. Endometrial biopsy alone is not an adequate method for excluding endometrial malignancy in higher risk groups.

Ultrasound Transvaginal scanning can be used to measure the double layer of endometrial thickness. In the largest study of ultrasound scan and PMB, nearly 1200 women were examined (Am J Obstet Gynecol 1995;172:1488). Using a cut-off of 4 mm, endometrial cancer was always detected but 5.5% of other endometrial pathology remained undetected. Fluid in the endometrial cavity on USS is associated with malignancy in 25% of cases. This was felt to compare favourably with dilatation and curettage.

PREMENSTRUAL SYNDROME

The incidence is 5–95% depending on the criteria used. It occurs more commonly in the multiparous woman, often after the first child.

Symptoms

More than 150 symptoms have been described. The character of the symptoms per se is not important, but they:

- should occur premenstrually,
- should be cyclical,
- should disappear or lessen after the onset of menstruation,
- should disrupt life,
- should be present for at least four out of six cycles.

Management

- Use a symptom calendar to establish the cyclical nature.
- Differentiate from major psychiatric disorders (especially bipolar illness), psychosexual problems, cyclical breast disorders, endometriosis, PID, PCOS, anaemia, thyroid dysfunction and the menopause (therefore consider Hb, TFTs, FSH and testosterone, if indicated).
- If there is serious diagnostic doubt, give goserelin 3.6 mg SC monthly for 3 months. Ignore symptoms of the first month, but any symptoms in the third month cannot be attributed to PMS.

Treatment

(There is a significant placebo effect, probably >50%.)

- Acknowledgement of the problem and reassurance may be all that are needed to enable the patient to cope. Are her partner and children understanding? Can she rearrange work schedules to reduce stress premenstrually?
- Fluoxetine (Prozac) at a dose of 20 mg/day is significantly superior to placebo in reducing symptoms of tension, irritability and dysphoria (N Engl J Med 1995;332:1574).
- Vitamin B_6 (pyridoxine) 50–100 mg/day may be effective. There is a risk of reversible peripheral neuropathy at high doses.
- Oil of evening primrose 4 × 500 mg capsules BD is expensive. Three small trials have shown improvement in mastalgia compared to placebo.
- Progestogens, (e.g. Provera 10 mg BD on days 12–26) have been tried. There have been many studies, none showing any benefit over placebo, although it may act as a minor tranquilliser.
- The low-dose COC may be worth an empirical trial in the low-risk patient, but benefits are unproven.
- Bromocriptine 5 mg/day on days 10–26 relieves cyclical breast symptoms, but has little effect on other symptoms. Many are unable to tolerate side-effects, however, with nausea and vomiting occurring in 50%. There may also be postural hypotension.
- Danazol 100 mg/day BD or QID is useful for breast symptoms, irritability, anxiety and lethargy. The side-effects are weight gain, acne, hirsutism, cramps, headaches and breast atrophy (if severe).

- Diuretics, e.g. spironolactone 25–50 mg/day for 7 days prior to menstruation, have been used for 'fluid retention'. There is no rational basis unless there is a proven premenstrual weight gain.
- GnRH agonists are a radical option, but they are expensive and lead to both flushings and hypo-oestrogenic problems, particularly osteoporosis.
- Oophorectomy (either laparoscopically or abdominally ± hysterectomy) is also a radical solution.

Some women find self-help groups supportive. General health measures (e.g. improved diet, reducing smoking and drinking, increased exercise, self-relaxation) often help. Herbal remedies are not scientifically tested, but some find them helpful (e.g. sage and fennel for irritability; rosemary, camomile and dandelion for breast tenderness). Women may also benefit from yoga, hypnosis, homeopathy or acupuncture.

PROLAPSE

> Cystourethrocele is the most common prolapse, followed by uterine descent and rectocele. A urethrocele occurring on its own is rare. An enterocele is more common following abdominal hysterectomy, vaginal hysterectomy or colposuspension. Symptoms do not necessarily depend on the size of the prolapse. Treatment may be conservative or surgical (Fig. 5.6).

Conservative treatment

Pessaries These are useful in those who are pregnant, or as a therapeutic test to confirm that surgery would be of benefit, or in those unfit or unwilling to undergo surgery. Ring pessaries are made of inert plastic and will give good vaginal wall support, providing that the perineum is sufficiently firm posteriorly to hold the ring in situ. The ring rests in the posterior fornix and sits over the symphysis pubis anteriorly (if fitting a ring on the first occasion, choose one with a diameter approximately equal to the posterior fornix–symphysis distance as estimated by a digital examination). A shelf-pessary is useful for uterine prolapse. Rings should be removed every 6–12 months, the vault inspected for inflammation or ulceration, and a new ring replaced. Short courses of topical vaginal oestrogens are occasionally required.

Surgical treatment

Cystocele Prolapse of the bladder (± urethra) may lead to discomfort, the feeling of 'something coming down' or urinary symptoms, particularly stress incontinence. Urgency and frequency are associated with cystocele and may (but do not necessarily) improve following surgery. A cystocele may also

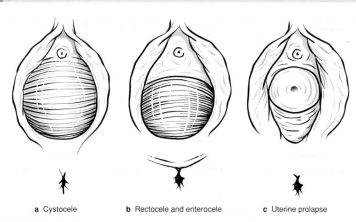

a Cystocele   **b** Rectocele and enterocele   **c** Uterine prolapse

Fig. 5.6 Vaginal wall prolapse.

cause obstruction, leading to urinary retention and overflow incontinence. Surgical correction of cystocele may be by anterior colporrhaphy (anterior repair) in which the vaginal skin is divided in the midline, the bladder (and urethra if there is a urethrocele) reflected upwards and the pubocervical fascia on either side buttressed with interrupted sutures. Redundant vaginal skin is excised and the vaginal epithelium closed. Postoperative urinary retention is common, and so a urethral or suprapubic catheter should be used. Burch colposuspension will also correct a cystocele and is more effective in improving stress incontinence (see p. 229).

Uterus and cervix This may cause low backache, often relieved by lying flat. It is graded as first degree (there is some descent within the vagina), second degree (the cervix appears at the introitus) or third degree or procidentia (the uterus is completely outside the vagina). With a procidentia, there may be ulceration, bleeding or an offensive discharge. Correction is by vaginal hysterectomy ±anterior or posterior repair. A Manchester repair (cervical amputation with anterior and posterior repair) probably also has a role in first- and second-degree prolapse.

Enterocele and vault prolapse These contain peritoneum and usually the small bowel or omentum. Enteroceles are repaired by opening the vaginal wall in the midline and dissecting the enterocele sac free, ligating it and closing the vaginal wall. Vault prolapse, traditionally treated by an abdominal colposacropexy (a non-absorbable mesh is used to join the vault to the anterior longitudinal ligament over the first sacral vertebra), may be more easily managed with a vaginal sacrospinous ligament fixation (the vault is supported by a stitch through the sacrospinous ligament, usually on just one side) (Br J Obstet Gynaecol 1998:13). This latter procedure probably carries a higher failure rate.

Rectocele This may give rise to backache, a lump in the vagina and a feeling of incomplete bowel emptying. The patient may be having to press the rectocele upwards at the time of defecation, or may be having to use digital evacuation. A vertical posterior vaginal wall incision is used to dissect the levator ani muscles and rectum. The levator ani muscles are sutured to the superficial perineal muscles, the redundant vaginal skin excised and the incision closed. It is easy to leave the vagina too narrow, and therefore only a little skin should be excised.

SECONDARY AMENORRHOEA

This is defined as no menstruation for 6 months (or ≥ three times the previous cycle length) in the absence of pregnancy. The commonest causes are weight loss, hyperprolactinaemia and PCOS.

Initial management

- Exclude pregnancy.
- Ask about perimenopausal symptoms (e.g. flushings, vaginal dryness).
- Take a history, including weight changes, drugs, medical disorders and thyroid symptoms.
- Carry out an examination looking particularly at height, weight, visual fields and the presence of hirsutism or virilization. Also carry out a pelvic examination (unless virgo intacta).
- Check serum for LH, FSH, Prl, testosterone, T_4 and TSH.
- Arrange a transvaginal USS; look for polycystic ovaries.
- Review back in the clinic with the results.

Further management

Ultrasound scan A scan showing multiple (>8) small, peripherally placed follicular ovarian cysts surrounded by a thickened echodense stroma confirms the diagnosis of polycystic ovaries. The diagnosis is supported by an LH:FSH ratio >3 and a testosterone level >3 mmol/l (see PCOS, p. 182).

Elevated prolactin level The Prl is >800 mU/l on at least two occasions (see hyperprolactinaemia, p. 184).

Elevated FSH (>30 U/l). Repeat the sample 6 weeks later. If FSH is still elevated and the patient >40 years old, the patient is menopausal (see p. 199). If the patient is <40 years old, the diagnosis is premature ovarian failure. This occurs in 1% of women and may be due to surgery, viral infections (e.g. mumps), cytotoxic drugs or radiotherapy. It may also be idiopathic, and is occasionally associated with chromosomal abnormality (XO mosaics or XXX). A low oestrogen level, very high FSH and the absence of any menstrual activity are poor prognostic signs for recovery. A biopsy is generally not indicated, as the histological correlation with prognosis is poor. Treat with HRT. Pregnancy by IVF with donor oocytes is possible. There is an association with other autoimmune disorders, so check antiovarian antibodies, FBC (? pernicious anaemia) and thyroid function.

Abnormal TFTs If the TFTs are abnormal, treat as appropriate.

If the above tests are normal, consider the following:

Weight loss The weight usually needs to be more than 45 kg, or the BMI (weight (kg)/height (m^2)) (see Appendix 6) greater than 17 for menstruation to occur. Loss of 10–15% weight usually leads to amenorrhoea. Anorexia nervosa is rare, with an incidence probably less than 1%. It can develop prior to menarche, is usually lifelong and is characterized by loss of insight regarding the distorted body image. There is loss of hair, increased lanugo, decreased pulse, lowered BP, anaemia, low basal LH and FSH and low oestrogen. Ovulation induction is possible with clomiphene or pulsatile GnRH in those wishing to conceive, but there is a much increased risk of fetal loss, IUGR and premature labour, so that it is ideal to wait until weight is restored spontaneously. Return of menstrual function may not be until months after the weight has been restored. The prevalence of bulimia is ≈1% and of these 60% will have had an episode of amenorrhoea at some time.

Depression, emotional disturbance and extreme exercise These may lead to amenorrhoea.

Sheehan syndrome Necrosis of the anterior pituitary following severe PPH is now very rare in the UK. It presents with failure of lactation, apathy, loss of axillary and pubic hair with symptoms and signs of hypothyroidism and adrenocortical insufficiency.

Asherman syndrome Secondary amenorrhoea following destruction of the endometrium by curettage is also relatively rare. Multiple synechiae are seen at hysteroscopy. Treatment involves breaking down the adhesions through a hysteroscope ±inserting an IUCD to deter reformation.

Idiopathic amenorrhoea This is sometimes called euoestrogenic amenorrhoea and usually responds well to clomiphene if fertility is required.

SEXUAL HEALTH

Sexual dysfunction is a common symptom in the gynaecology clinic, and patients' ability to share their problem often depends on the attitude of the clinician. Simple, open-ended questions asked in a relaxed, non-judgmental atmosphere will be rewarded. The possibility of sexual dysfunction should be particularly borne in mind in infertility and colposcopy clinics, after gynaecological surgery (especially for cancer) and in those on medication (anticholinergics, antidepressants, spironolactone, cimetidine, steroids, antihypertensives). (ABC of sexual health, Br Med J, 1999)

The history should include the problem as the patient sees it, how long the problem has been present and whether the problem is related to the time, place or partner. It is also important to establish whether there is a loss of sex drive or dislike of sexual contact, or whether there are problems within the relationship. Consider whether there is anxiety, guilt or anger which is not being expressed, and enquire about whether there are physical problems (e.g. pain) with either partner. A social history is appropriate and medical history essential (depression, diabetes, osteoarthritis).

It is good practice to offer to have a chaperone present for both male and female patients if they wish. (A substantial minority of patients, both men and women, prefer to be examined by a doctor of their own sex (remember that patients have made complaints of indecent assault, even when their examining doctor was of the same sex). Cultural differences must also be considered. Many Muslim, Hindu and Sikh women practise a strict sexual morality. Girls are brought up to be shy and modest, and submitting to a vaginal examination may be regarded with abhorrence, even as a matter of life and death. Remember that your own sexual mores may not be universally accepted.

Examination is necessary when a physical problem is suspected and may not always be appropriate. In the female patient assess the development of secondary sexual characteristics and exclude hirsutism or other signs of virilization. Check the BP, radial pulse and urine. Examine the abdomen and the reflexes, including a check of the anal reflex if a neurological problem is suspected. Digital and speculum examination of the vagina may be appropriate to exclude congenital abnormalities, infection, episiotomy scarring, uterine tenderness and adnexal pathology. Endocrine investigation has limited role but LH, FSH, T_4, Prl and testosterone may be relevant. Genital and systemic examinations in the male may also be appropriate, looking particularly for gynaecomastia, and testing for tactile (dorsal column) and pinprick (spinothalamic tract) sensation in the perineal and lower limb dermatomes. Check urinalysis for sugar.

FEMALE

Dyspareunia

This is common and may be due to organic pathology. The pain may be reproducible during VE. It may be superficial (e.g. infection, Bartholin's gland cyst, episiotomy scars) or deep (e.g. endometriosis, chronic PID, ovarian cysts, large fibroids, retroverted uterus). Frequently, however, examination (which may include laparoscopy) is normal. Vaginismus, poor lubrication and penetration before arousal are common causes of dyspareunia. There may be help with the use of different positions. If the vagina is dry, a lubricating gel (e.g. KY Jelly) ± HRT perimenopausally may be of help.

Vaginismus

This is characterized by involuntary spasm of the pubococcygeus muscle such that penetration is difficult or impossible. It may begin after a minor episode of pain (e.g. due to thrush) and occur on subsequent occasions before penetration to prevent the painful episode happening again. This makes penetration more painful and so the cycle continues, being further exacerbated by anxiety. Vaginismus may be related to personality, sexual attitudes or the ability to become aroused. Speculum and vaginal examination may be impossible. Vaginismus is best treated by using graded vaginal dilators with regular supervision and encouragement (±sensate focus, see p. 215) and Kegel exercises to allow voluntary relaxation of the pubococcygeus.

Orgasmic dysfunction

This may be associated with general sexual dysfunction. If it occurs despite achieving arousal, it is best managed with instruction in masturbatory techniques.

General sexual dysfunction

This is lack of sexual interest or arousal. It is often associated with guilt, self-blame and at times positive avoidance of sex. Ask about symptoms of depression or anxiety. Remember that breast-feeding is a powerful cause of lack of sex drive (due to high prolactin levels).

MALE

Erectile difficulty

Penile erection is due to relaxation of the smooth muscle around the cavernosal vascular spaces, allowing them to fill with blood. This is under the control of the autonomic nervous system, mediated by cyclic guanosine monophosphate (cGMP). Erectile failure is common, with 52% of men aged 40–70 years suffering the problem to some degree. As approximately 75% will have an organic component, drug treatment is now often used in addition to, or instead of, psychosexual counselling.

Treatment
Treatment options include the following:

Sildenafil (Viagra) This drug is taken orally and acts as an enhancer of erection by blocking breakdown of cGMP. It works best in psychogenic erectile failure and milder organic problems in which the success rate is ≈85%. Side-effects are mild and transient and include flushing, dyspepsia, headache and transient disturbance in colour vision (N Engl J Med 1998;May:338). It must not be used with nitrates (may lead to a potentially life-threatening profound drop in BP).

Alprostadil (PGE₁) This drug also relaxes cavernosal smooth muscle but must be injected directly into the corpora cavernosa. It is more effective than sildenafil in erectile failure due to more severe organic problems. It is also available as a urethral pellet (MUSE) but this is much less effective.

Other treatments These include vacuum devices and penile implants, the latter only being suitable where no other treatment has been effective.

Ejaculatory problems

Premature ejaculation may be defined as the tendency to ejaculate too quickly for his own, or his partner's, satisfaction. Delayed ejaculation is the reverse and is more difficult to treat. Retrograde ejaculation occurs when the seminal fluid passes backwards into the bladder (e.g. postprostatectomy, spinal cord injury). A man with premature ejaculation can learn to delay his ejaculation by means of a programme of graded masturbatory exercises (the squeeze technique). Intercourse should proceed as usual until ejaculation is felt to be inevitable. The couple should then stop and either the man or his partner should squeeze just below the glans penis. This is repeated four or five times before ejaculation is allowed to occur. Fluoxetine 20 mg/day on days when intercourse is planned often helps in severe cases.

Reduced sexual desire

As in the female, this is poorly understood, but may be related to upbringing, poor social skills, lack of opportunity or lack of sexual education. Increased Prl is a rare cause, and some men aged >50 years have decreased testosterone due to testicular failure and may require testosterone replacement.

TREATMENT FOR THE COUPLE

It is important to exclude organic pathology, and laparoscopy may be warranted, particularly in dyspareunia. The routine gynaecology clinic is an inappropriate setting for a series of long consultations (unless at the end of the clinic) and continuity with one counsellor is crucial. Consider referral to a sexual dysfunction clinic. Both partners should attend, as they usually both contribute to problems.

Management

In some instances, reassurance or information may be all that is required. Patients often want to check that their sexual practice is normal (e.g. positions used, oral sex, lights on/off). This includes confirming that it is acceptable to be less sexually active (e.g. in the puerperium or postmenopausally) or may apply to sexual orientation. Although our society encourages discussion about sexuality, there is still ignorance and naiveté in some couples (e.g. they are unaware that the rate of arousal is faster in males than in females and that penetration before the female is aroused will result in pain from dryness and failure of ballooning of the vagina).

Also note that:

- most women are more likely to achieve orgasm by masturbation, partner digital stimulation of clitoris or oral sex than by intercourse;
- most women do not experience multiple orgasms;
- women may initiate sex;
- intercourse is not essential (unless fertility is required);
- masturbation (including using a vibrator) is neither dirty nor harmful;
- if a man loses his erection, it does not mean he does not find his partner attractive;
- reduced libido is common in pregnancy and the puerperium.

The following books may be of help to patients:

- D. Delvin, *The book of love*, revised edn., New England Library, 1992.
- *The mature couple's guide to love and intimacy*. In the series *Sex, a lifelong pleasure*. Visual corporation, London (Tel: 01371 873 138).
- *Lovers' guide*. A series introduced by Dr Andrew Stanway, Carlton Home Entertainment, London (Tel: 0208 207 6207).

Intensive therapy Dyspareunia (without identifiable cause), the orgasmic dysfunctions and the male dysfunctions may be treated with a behavioural approach (e.g. 12 fortnightly consultations). This treatment (sensate focus) consists of a programme of tasks that a couple can undertake in their own time at home. Underlying the programme is a ban on sexual intercourse or any genital contact until anxiety about performance and fear of failure have subsided and trust between the couple has been established. This ban ensures that physical intimacy will not lead to sexual intimacy. The tasks involve the couple setting aside time to explore each other's bodies in turn by touching, stroking, caressing and massaging, gradually introducing sensual, then erotic, and then sexual touch over a period of time. About two-thirds will be 'much improved', although there is a significant long-term recurrence rate. Once again, this is best carried out in a specific clinic rather than by generalists in a gynaecology setting.

Sensate focus

Stage 1
1. Taking plenty of time, each partner explores the other's naked (if possible) body, avoiding breasts and genitals, avoiding trying to give pleasure, and concentrating on feelings and sensations experienced in both 'active' and 'passive' roles.
2. After 2 weeks or 4 sessions of this, some familiarity and trust should allow inclusion of breasts and experimentation with a variety of touches, such as with body oils, talcum powder, feathers, fabrics, etc.
3. As above, but adding the making of specific requests for preferred types of touch and the use of a back-to-front position to enable the person being touched to guide the partner's hand.

Stage 2
1. Maintain the ban on intercourse, but include genital touching as part of the established exercises, so there are now no forbidden areas.
2. While continuing all the above, concentrate more on the genitals to discover the sensations resulting from different pressures in different areas.
3. This is an optional stage for mutual masturbation to orgasm.

Stage 3
1. While continuing all the above and maintaining the ban on full intercourse, the next step is containment without movement, allowing the penis to be accepted and contained by the vagina (modified for homosexual couples). Couples should progress at their preferred pace.
2. Containment with gentle thrusting and rotating movement.
3. Thrusting to orgasm.

The couple need to be monitored to agree the ground rules and the staged tasks, to deal with any issues that may arise as a result of the tasks, to support positive changes and to prevent relapse in the early stages. Suggested ground rules are:

- Agree a ban on sexual intercourse and genital touching.
- Set up twice-weekly times to spend on this homework, increasing from 20 minutes to 60 minutes over 4 weeks.
- During these times, speak only if the partner's touch is painful or unacceptable. Otherwise it is assumed that what is being done is all right. Conversation will prevent concentration on the task and render it pointless.
- Attention should be focused on personal experience, not on pleasing the partner. This is a learning exercise above all.

SURGERY IN GYNAECOLOGY

> This section is not intended as a surgical textbook and is simply a guide for those beginning their surgical experience to appreciate the sequence of events in a few selected basic procedures. It is in no way a substitute for experienced practical teaching, and surgery must not be undertaken without appropriate supervision.

PREOPERATIVE CONSIDERATIONS

> - Does the patient need the operation – have alternatives been considered and discussed (e.g. see alternatives to surgery for menorrhagia, p. 203)?
> - Make sure the patient is not pregnant.

Consent
See particularly page 258. Some areas of controversy are highlighted below:

Sterilization
See page 170, and ensure that all the points covered have been fully documented.

TABLE 5.9	**Advantages and disadvantages of different hysterectomy methods**	
Method	*Advantages*	*Disadvantages*
Total abdominal hysterectomy	The cervix is removed and therefore no further smears are required and there is no risk of cervical malignancy (therefore this is particularly suitable for those with a history of abnormal cytology). Good access to ovaries	Increased surgical morbidity. The cervix is considered by some to have a role in sexual function
Subtotal abdominal hysterectomy	Fewer complications than total abdominal hysterectomy (↓bleeding, ↓infection, ↓bladder injury, ↓ureteric damage). Good access to ovaries	The risk of cervical cancer remains as before
Vaginal hysterectomy	Lower incidence of bladder and bowel injury in straightforward cases (compared to abdominal hysterectomy). No potentially painful abdominal wound	There is only limited ovarian access. Is contraindicated with: • large uterus • restricted uterine mobility • limited vaginal space • adnexal pathology • cervix flush with vagina

Choice of abdominal vs vaginal hysterectomy (Table 5.9)

Subtotal hysterectomy carries a lower morbidity than a total abdominal hysterectomy – there is less bleeding and fewer wound and urine infections and a lower incidence of urinary tract damage. Vaginal hysterectomy is probably superior to the abdominal approach in appropriate cases in that there is no abdominal wound and there is also a lower incidence of bladder, ureteric and bowel injury. Laparoscopically assisted procedures are not discussed here.

Normal ovaries at abdominal hysterectomy

The decision of whether to remove ovaries at abdominal hysterectomy depends on the patient's wishes, her age, her family history of breast or ovarian carcinoma (see p. 251) and her plans for HRT (see p. 200). In a 50-year-old woman, it is unlikely that there will be much further ovarian function (average age of menopause 51 years), and bilateral salpingo-oophorectomy will significantly reduce the incidence of later ovarian carcinoma. Residual ovaries may also occasionally cause chronic pain or dyspareunia if adherent to the posterior fornix. In a 40-year-old woman, however, a further 10 years of ovarian oestrogen secretion may be expected. It is unclear whether HRT is as effective in terms of long-term prophylaxis as endogenous oestrogens. It may therefore be appropriate to discuss routine oophorectomy in those aged over 45 and ovarian conservation in those under 45. The decision must remain, however, a very individualized consideration.

Bladder, bowel and sexual dysfunction after hysterectomy (Br J Obstet Gynaecol 1997:983)

There is conflicting evidence about whether abdominal hysterectomy has any effect on bladder function (there have been no studies looking at vaginal hysterectomy and urinary dysfunction). The picture is just as confused with bowel function. With regard to sexual dysfunction, it is probable that women who retain an overall normal sexual desire have improved postoperative satisfaction, presumably because in some instances painful pathology has been reduced.

Antibiotic prophylaxis

There is evidence that the use of single or short courses of broad-spectrum antibiotics at the time of major surgery reduces the incidence of postoperative infection. Screening for chlamydia ±antibiotic prophylaxis for those aged <30 years undergoing uterine instrumentation may also be appropriate.

Venous thromboembolic prophylaxis

Venous thromboembolic disease accounts for around 20% of perioperative hysterectomy deaths. As prophylaxis is effective in reducing thromboembolism (Table 5.10), all gynaecological patients should be assessed for risk factors and prophylaxis prescribed accordingly (Table 5.11). The incidence is higher

TABLE 5.10 Meta-analysis of incidence of deep venous thrombosis after major general surgery (defined by ^{125}I scanning)

Prophylaxis	Mean incidence (%)
No prophylaxis	25
Low-dose heparin	9
Graduated elastic compression stockings	9
Intermittent pneumatic compression	10
Dextran	17
Aspirin	20

in those with malignancy (35%), lower for 'routine' abdominal hysterectomy (12%) and lowest for vaginal hysterectomy.

As some prophylactic methods may be associated with side-effects (e.g. wound haematomas, hypersensitivity reactions with heparin) the methods

TABLE 5.11 Risk factors given as % for venous thromboembolic disease*

Risk group	Details	Deep venous thrombosis	Proximal vein thrombosis	Fatal pulmonary embolism	Suggestion for prophylaxis
Low	Minor surgery (<30 min); no risk factors other than age Major surgery (<30 min); age <40 years; no other risk factors (as below)	<10	<1	0.01	Early mobilization ± graduated compression stockings
Moderate	Minor surgery (<30 min) with personal or family history of DVT, PE or thrombophilia Major gynaecological surgery (>30 min) Age >40 years, obesity (>80 kg), gross varicose veins, current infection Immobility prior to surgery (>4 days) Major medical illness: heart or lung disease, cancer, inflammatory bowel disease	10–40	1–10	0.1–1	Early mobilization ± graduated compression stockings + heparin (e.g. 5000 U SC BD or enoxaparin 20 mg/day)
High	Three or more of above risk factors Major pelvic or abdominal surgery for cancer Major surgery in patients with previous DVT, pulmonary embolism, thrombophilia, or lower limb paralysis (e.g. hemiplegic stroke, paraplegia)	40–80	10–30	1–10	Early mobilization ± graduated compression stockings + heparin (e.g. 5000 U SC TID or enoxaparin 40 mg/day)

(*Incidences based on Br Med J 1992;305:567; suggested prophylaxis based on RCOG Working Party 1995)

chosen must be based on some form of risk vs benefit assessment. The benefits to the patient of heparin in moderate/high risk groups are felt to outweigh the approximately 2:100 risk of wound haematoma, which may be minimized by avoiding injection close to the wound. Graduated compression stockings would be an alternative, although compliance with stockings may be reduced in those who find them uncomfortable. In addition, they have not been shown to reduce the risk of fatal pulmonary thromboembolism. Dextran carries a significant risk of anaphylaxis.

Any benefits to stopping the COC 4–6 weeks prior to surgery must be weighed against the risk of unwanted pregnancy. In the absence of other risk factors there is insufficient evidence to support a policy of routine COC discontinuation. It is probably not necessary to stop HRT for surgery.

SPECIFIC SURGICAL CONSIDERATIONS

Assisting and operating

> Cut well, tie well, get well! (Denton Cooley, Pioneer Cardiac Transplant Surgeon)

It is important to master good technique at the start, as bad habits are hard to lose. Practice releasing clamps slowly and steadily with each hand. Use forceps and scissors with your hands supinated (allows a better view of the end of the instrument). Ask someone who can tie knots properly to show you how, and practice single and double throws, ensuring that each throw is tied in the opposite direction to the one below it. The knots should be tightened with the index or middle fingers pulling in opposite directions (otherwise there is tension on the structure being tied rather than on the knot itself).

Ask for the lights to be arranged to maximal benefit. Stand on two feet, not one. Lean your hips against the table for support (not your elbows on the patient's chest). If making an incision, apply even tension to the skin to allow a cleaner cut. If swabbing out, try not to traumatize visceral structures or tied pedicles, which may make bleeding worse. If there is deep venous bleeding, it is often easier to identify the site using suction rather than swabs. It is well worth reading traditional accounts of the fine points of theatre technique, (e.g. Bonney's gynaecological surgery, Cassell, London).

EUA, dilatation and curettage ± hysteroscopy

Place the patient in the lithotomy position. Inspect the vulva. If a smear is required, do this before washing and draping. Carry out a thorough EUA, noting uterine size, shape, mobility and the presence of adnexal masses (it is usually possible to feel normal ovaries unless the patient is obese). Insert a Sims' speculum and grasp the anterior lip of the cervix with at least one volsellum. Check for uterine descent and lateral access (i.e. suitability for vaginal hysterectomy if this is ever required). Insert a uterine sound gently, taking care that the angulation of the curve is in the direction of the uterine cavity (i.e. concave anteriorly for an anteverted uterus) and measure to the cavity length. Beware of creating a false passage or perforating the uterine fundus (it helps to hold a finger on the sound and dilators to prevent sudden slippage). If perforation occurs, abandon the procedure and give antibiotics. If the uterus was perforated with a sound or small dilator, conservative management is probably appropriate. If perforation was with a suction curette or grasping forceps the risk of bowel injury is much higher, and laparoscopy or laparotomy should be considered.

The extent of dilatation depends on the instrument to be inserted (e.g. 5–6 mm for a 5 mm hysteroscope, 5–10 mm for a curette, and approximately the number of weeks of gestation for TOP or ERPOC, usually 8, 10 or 12 weeks being 8, 10 or 12 mm). A hysteroscope can use fluid (e.g. Hartman's solution) or CO_2 to insufflate the cavity. After inspection of the cavity and both ostia it is common to curette radially to obtain an endometrial sample (e.g. at 10, 2, 5 and 7 o'clock, or at any specific area thought to be suspicious at hysteroscopy). ERPOC or suction TOP up to 12 weeks is best performed with suction through either a flexible or a rigid curette (see p. 155). A balance needs to be struck between excessive curettage, which might lead to Asherman's syndrome, and leaving tissue behind (an empty uterus has a sandpaper feel on curettage).

Laparoscopy

Place the patient in the Lloyd Davis position. Ensure asepsis. Empty the bladder, unless you are certain that patient has voided just prior to theatre. Instrument the uterus only if you are certain that there is no intrauterine pregnancy. After putting the patient's head downwards, insufflate the abdomen with CO_2. This can either be done blind (Veress needle inserted subumbilically and aimed towards the coccyx to avoid the aortic bifurcation, or suprapubically aimed posteriorly) or under direct vision after cut-down, particularly if there are concerns about adhesions. Check that the flow rate is normal and that the abdomen is distending *symmetrically* and becoming resonant. After insufflating ≈2 litres of gas the needle is removed and a trochar inserted for the telescope ± camera. All subsequent ports should be under direct intra-abdominal vision by telescope. Midline ports have a much lower associated incidence of Richter's herniae and midline entry also minimizes the risk of injury to the inferior epigastric artery (runs from the external iliac artery upwards, anterior to the arcuate ligament and then between the posterior lamina of the rectus sheath and posterior aspect of rectus abdominis). Carry out a thorough inspection of pelvic organs, including lifting the ovaries to check the ovarian fossae. If tubal function is being assessed, inject dilute methylene blue through the cervical cannulae and inspect the fimbrial end of each tube. If PID is suspected, check the liver (? peri-hepatic adhesions, p. 190).

At the end, release the gas. Some clinicians leave ports to heal spontaneously while others suture the skin. Lateral ports >10 mm carry a high risk of Richter's herniae and should have the sheath and skin closed, care being taken not to include viscera in the stitch (there are a number of specialized techniques for this).

Abdominal hysterectomy

This may be carried out using a lower abdominal transverse incision (as for caesarean section, see p. 90) or, if the uterus is large or there are large ovarian cysts, through a midline or paramedian incision. If malignancy is suspected, take saline washings on opening the peritoneum, and palpate the paracolic gutters, liver and diaphragm. Place two clamps just lateral to the uterus on either side over the round and broad ligaments (Fig. 5.7), taking care to leave the tips well short of the bladder. Angle the tips slightly outwards into the broad ligament to avoid cutting the ascending uterine artery just lateral to the uterine body. If taking the ovary, clamp the round ligament laterally and divide it to open up the leaves of the broad ligament. Taking a finger posteriorly, press it through the posterior leaf of the broad ligament lateral to the ovary (i.e. under the infundibulopelvic ligament) and push it up to the space in the divided round ligament. Clamp the infundibulopelvic ligament, taking care that it does not contain the ureter as it crosses the pelvic brim (this is usually a problem only if anatomy is distorted, e.g. by severe endometriosis or a large ovarian cyst). Divide medial to the clamp. This and the lateral part of the round ligament should be tied and may be double tied together for extra security. Repeat on the other side. If the ovaries are not

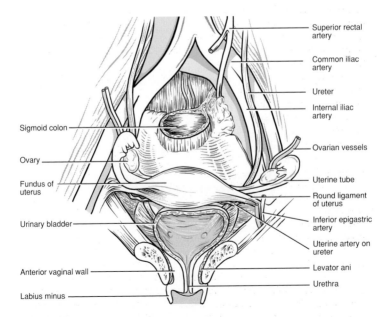

Fig. 5.7 Pelvic anatomy – anterior view.

being taken it is usually possible to draw the ovary laterally (one finger in front and the other behind the broad ligament) and place a second clamp medial to the ovary, with the point almost touching the initial clamp. The round and ovarian ligaments can then be divided and tied together.

Open the uterovesical peritoneum by lifting with dissecting forceps and dividing with scissors, starting from the already partially opened broad ligament laterally. This allows the bladder to be pushed downwards, either with a swab or by freeing it with scissors, care being taken to keep the scissor points pointing posteriorly away from the bladder. If in the wrong plane (usually too superficial) there may be a lot of troublesome bleeding from the venous plexus behind the bladder. The lateral angles of the bladder need to be given attention to ensure that the ureters are clear. Also, palpate to ensure that the ureter is out of the way before clamping each uterine artery and ligating the pedicles. Particular care of the ureter is required in the presence of fibroids or endometriosis.

There are many different ways to complete the operation. The top of the vagina may be opened in the midline with a scalpel, cutting laterally with scissors to clamp the cardinal and uterosacral ligaments before continuing round to the back of the vagina. Alternatively, these ligaments can be clamped initially, working downwards to the vaginal vault before opening the vagina to remove the uterus. Throughout, care is necessary to avoid damage to bladder, ureters and bowel. The vault can be closed with an interrupted or continuous suture.

Vaginal hysterectomy

Grasp the cervix (Fig. 5.8) with volsellum forceps and pull down. Circumcise it all the way around, allowing the bladder to be reflected upwards anteriorly (opening the uterovesical pouch at this point if possible). The pouch of Douglas should be visualized posteriorly. Open the pouch with scissors, widen it digitally and clamp the uterosacral ± the cardinal ligaments laterally. Dividing and tying these allows the uterine arteries to be clamped and divided, and access obtained to the broad ligament, round ligament and fallopian tube. These can then also be clamped and divided. Throughout, keep as close into the uterus as possible to avoid injury to more lateral structures. With a larger uterus, or where access is more difficult, it is often necessary to take multiple pedicles on each side rather than the four described.

After ensuring haemostasis there are a number of ways to close, but the uterosacral and cardinal ligaments are often sutured into the vault to provide support. The vault itself is then closed with continuous or interrupted sutures.

Anterior colporrhaphy

Grasp the cervix with volsellum forceps and pull down. Consider injecting 10–20 ml of 0.5% bupivacaine with 1:200 000 adrenaline superficially to the cystocele to aid haemostasis. Make a small transverse incision above the

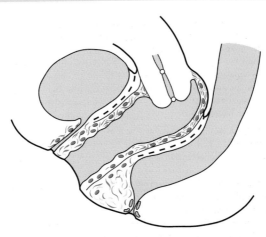

Fig. 5.8 Vagina, cervix and uterus – lateral view. The barred lines (— — — —) define the avascular areolar planes between the thick vascular vaginal walls and the bladder (anteriorly), and the rectum (posteriorly). These planes extend up to the peritoneal reflexions. Note: below the bladder neck and the apex of the perineal body, there are no natural planes of separation.

cervix but below the bladder, and attach two small clips to the upper lip of this. It is then possible to run a pair of curved scissors (points upwards) into the relatively avascular plane between the vaginal mucosa and the bladder, allowing division of the mucosa in the midline. This is held laterally while the bladder is reflected, care being taken to ensure that the reflection is started as far laterally as possible to avoid bladder damage and that it is reflected in the avascular plane. The bladder is then pushed well upwards.

Two or three buttressing sutures are placed as deeply as possible into the lateral fascia, redundant skin is excised in the midline and the full thickness of vaginal wall reapposed with interrupted sutures.

Posterior colporrhaphy

Incise the posterior fourchette transversely for 1–2 cm and grasp the upper lip of the incision with two small clips. As for the anterior colporrhaphy, use curved scissors to identify the avascular plane between the vagina and rectum and divide the vaginal skin vertically in the midline. Again, use sharp and blunt dissection to push the bowel laterally, free of the vaginal skin on each side. Buttress the fascia on each side with interrupted sutures before excising redundant skin (take care in posterior vaginal surgery not to excise too much skin) and close with a continuous or interrupted suture.

If there is also an enterocele, it is necessary to extend the incision upwards over this, opening the sac of peritoneum, reducing the contents and ligating it as high as possible before reclosing.

Course of the ureter

The ureter runs a retroperitoneal course from the renal pelvis downwards and slightly medially over psoas major, entering the pelvis over the external iliac artery and vein. It runs down over the anterior branch of the internal iliac artery and follows the anterior border of the greater sciatic notch until, opposite the ischial spine, it turns anteromedially into the fascia of the lower part of the broad ligament. It then continues medially towards the cervix. Two centimetres lateral to the cervix it is crossed by the uterine artery before turning anteriorly to the base of the bladder. The uterine artery in turn reaches the side of the uterus and ascends to anastomose with the ovarian artery from above as well as sending branches downwards to the cervix and vagina.

POST OPERATIVE CONSIDERATIONS

 Check that thromboprophylactic measures are appropriate.

The most likely complication in the first 24 postoperative hours is haemorrhage. If there are significant signs of haemorrhage (blood in drain, pale patient, increased pulse, decreased BP, distending pale abdomen) it may often be necessary to return to theatre. Experienced surgical help should be sought. Site two IV infusions, crossmatch 6 u RCC, check clotting, and involve the anaesthetist early.

In the routine postoperative days, check the patient's general appearance, and look for pyrexia, abdominal pain and distension, and urinary or bowel difficulties. If the haemoglobin has fallen, consider whether the loss in theatre was sufficient to account for the drop, or whether there might be a haematoma (pain, pyrexia, delayed restoration of bowel sounds and, occasionally, urinary retention). Management is often conservative unless problems are severe.

If the patient is pyrexial, are there symptoms or signs to suggest UTI, DVT or chest infection? Send an MSU sample for analysis. Note that 50% of DVTs have no demonstrable clinical signs (see DVT Management, p. 147). Abdominal distension may be the result of a haematoma (as above), postoperative ileus or true bowel obstruction. Consider AXR if there is possible worsening bowel obstruction.

Discharge Try and ensure that the patient knows what has been done and why. What, if anything, happens next. What medication has been described and what follow-up is to be arranged (find out who is to make the appointment). Does the patient need to see the GP? Are there any results still to get? Who should the patient contact if there is a problem? If appropriate, ensure HRT has been started (see p. 200). Also, discuss resumption of activity, work and sex.

UROGYNAECOLOGY

URINARY INCONTINENCE

> Urinary incontinence is the involuntary loss of urine which is objectively demonstrated and is socially a problem.

The main causes of urinary incontinence are shown in Table 6.1.

TABLE 6.1 Causes of urinary incontinence

Cause	Approximate incidence in gynaecological population with incontinence
Genuine stress incontinence (GSI) due to urethral sphincter weakness	≥60%
The urge syndrome, combining motor urgency (primary detrusor instability (DI)), sensory urgency and extrinsic pathology	20–30% (70–80% in the geriatric population)
Mixed incontinence, usually a mixture of GSI and DI	20–30%
Fistulae, urethral obstruction with overflow (voiding difficulty), congenital anomalies, neurological disorders, diverticulae, dementia and others	5%

History

- Is there stress incontinence, urgency, urge incontinence, enuresis or continuous leakage?
- How much does it affect lifestyle (important when considering surgery)?
- Is sanitary protection used (e.g. change of underwear, towels, minipads, large pads)?
- Is fluid throughput thought to be high, average or low (normal ≈1500 ml/24 h)?
- Nocturia (once or twice is normal); frequency, urgency, urge incontinence, enuresis and adverse effect of running water are features of urge syndrome.
- Dysuria suggests cystitis.
- Is there incontinence with intercourse (leakage with penetration suggests stress incontinence and those with DI leak at orgasm)?
- Haematuria can indicate malignancy (particularly in older women), but more commonly infection.
- Pushing or straining to void (±absent sensation) suggests outflow obstruction or detrusor hypocontractility or acontractility.
- Drug history, particularly diuretics and psychotropics.
- Has any treatment been tried (pelvic exercises, drugs, operations)?

Frequency–volume chart This provides a simple, objective 3-day method of assessing a patient's bladder function and habit. A record is kept of the time and volume of each urination. A normal woman passes about 1500 ml/24 hours in 6–8 voids and the bladder capacity is usually (but not always) 300–500 ml. Any wide variation from this may indicate an abnormality (e.g. a total output of > 2000 ml is excessive unless there is a history of recurrent infection and an output < 1000 ml may predispose to infection). With DI, smaller volumes are passed more frequently day and night (e.g. 100–200 ml).

Clinical examination

- General examination. Is the patient obese?
- Pelvic examination:
  — Exclude a pelvic mass (may predispose to urgency).
  — Is there a good vaginal squeeze? (If fair or good, pelvic floor exercises should be of help. If weak, refer to the physiotherapist for supervised exercises ± electrical treatment). Ask the patient to cough.
  — Is there urinary leakage (confirms complaint)? Is there a cystocele (may predispose to GSI or obstruction with overflow)?
- Urinalysis for blood, sugar and protein. Send an MSU if positive.

Urodynamic investigations

These are indicated preoperatively, after failed surgery, for unusual symptoms, or in the presence of residual urine, recurrent infection or other abnormality (e.g. fistula). It may, for example, be important to differentiate GSI as a cause of stress incontinence from unstable detrusor contractions provoked by coughing. These investigations may not be universally available, however, and have a relatively low sensitivity and specificity. Some clinicians do not perform urodynamics on all preoperative patients with stress incontinence if there are no features in the history to suggest bladder instability.

Cystometry This is a method of assessing detrusor activity during a series of provocation tests such as with coughing, when voiding and on bladder filling. Intravesical pressure is composed of both transmitted abdominal pressure (e.g. coughing) and detrusor contraction pressure. Static cystometry therefore requires intravesical and intrarectal (= intra-abdominal) pressure lines and a urethral catheter to allow retrograde bladder filling. Detrusor activity may be observed by electronic subtraction or 'eyeballing' the record. After an initial independent flow rate to exclude obstruction, the residual volume is measured (normal <50–100 ml). The bladder is then filled and the first desire to void noted (usually around 200 ml; earlier suggests DI). The total capacity is noted (usually >400 ml; lower suggests DI). There should be no leakage with coughing (leakage in the absence of detrusor contraction indicates GSI), and no detrusor contractions during the filling phase until the patient is asked to void (contractions while the patient is trying to inhibit micturition suggests DI). Ambulatory cystometry is more time consuming, but may be more sensitive and specific (Neurol Urodynam 1997:510).

Videocystometry. (This is also known as *video pressure/flow cystometry*). This is used to observe bladder neck opening at rest or on coughing. It is also used to demonstrate leakage on provocation (e.g. coughing) and vesicoureteric reflux (e.g. patients with recurrent UTI).

Flow study This measures the rate of flow (normal >15 ml/s). The flow rate is reduced in outflow obstruction (uncommon in women).

USS This measures residual urine volume (useful if there is possible retention, e.g. postoperatively, postdelivery).

Cystoscopy and IVU These are particularly appropriate with haematuria in the elderly, with recurrent UTI and to exclude chronic cystitis, stones and tumours.

Electromyography This is required when neurological dysfunction is suspected.

GENUINE STRESS INCONTINENCE (GSI)

GSI is the involuntary loss of urine when intravesical pressure exceeds the maximum urethral closure pressure in the absence of detrusor activity. It is caused by either bladder neck hypermobility or intrinsic sphincter deficiency. Diagnosis is suggested by a history of leakage with coughing, laughing, sneezing or exercise, and may be supported by clinical examination and a frequency–volume chart. Cystometry may occasionally be required if there is diagnostic confusion, as the above stimuli may also provoke pathological detrusor contractions. Any benefit of this investigation remains unproven.

Conservative treatment for GSI
This is very effective in many patients and avoids the potentially serious complications of surgery. It should always be tried before considering surgery.

- Stop smoking (therefore less coughing) and lose weight.
- If mild, insertion of a tampon (e.g. before exercise) may be of help as a temporary measure.
- Pelvic floor exercises. The patient is advised to squeeze repeatedly (as if trying to stop the passage of flatus) for 2 minutes twice every day over a number of months. Alternatively 'cones', which are smooth graded tampon-like weights, can be inserted and held, the weight being increased as the muscle strength improves. These are preferable to midstream stops, which increase intravesical pressure and may lead to back-pressure on the kidneys.

- Electrical treatment to the vaginal muscles (e.g. interferential therapy). Pelvic floor exercises have been found to be more effective than electrical treatment or cones (Br Med J 1999;318:487).
- There is conflicting evidence concerning the effect of oestrogens in the postmenopausal patient.

Surgical treatment for GSI (Br J Obstet Gynaecol 1994:371)
The choice of operation depends on the surgeon's preference, the patient's general health, the degree of prolapse and previous surgery. A choice may have to be made between cure rate and morbidity (e.g. bladder-neck elevation vs periurethral bulking agents). Surgery aims to elevate the bladder neck, but the mechanism by which this confers benefit remains controversial. If the history is not one of pure GSI, cystometry should be carried out prior to surgery. Although traditional teaching is that elevation of the bladder neck exacerbates DI, objective studies with colposuspension suggest that DI is caused or cured in equal proportions.

Retropubic procedures

Burch colposuspension (Fig. 6.1) Through a pfannenstiel incision, the retropubic space is opened and the bladder neck identified. This is then suspended from the iliopectineal (Cooper's) ligaments by 2–4 sutures (e.g. PDS, Ethibond, Vicryl) on each side. The mean success rate is almost 90%, but 5–18% develop de novo detrusor instability and up to 18% may develop an enterocele or rectocele. There are postoperative voiding difficulties in ≈10%.

- Lloyd Davis pontion.
- low transverse incision
- Cave of Retzius
- urethral catheterisation to identify bladder neck
- SPC.

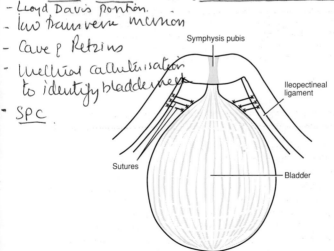

Symphysis pubis

Ileopectineal ligament

Sutures

Bladder

Fig. 6.1 The Burch colposuspension.

Marshall–Marchetti–Krantz procedure This is similar to the Burch procedure, with the bladder neck being supported instead from the periosteum on the symphysis pubis. The mean success rate and incidence of detrusor instability are similar to the colposuspension, but it will not correct a cystocele and there is the additional complication of osteitis pubis (2–5%) which is difficult to treat and may become chronic.

Tension-free vaginal tape In this relatively new procedure a specially designed Prolene tape is placed transvaginally, supporting the urethra in a tension-free manner, with the ends of the tape brought out through suprapubic stab incisions. Morbidity is claimed to be much reduced. (Intl Urogynaecol J Pelvic Floor Dysfunction 1997:8).

Needle suspension procedures

Pereyra A special long needle is inserted through two small suprapubic incisions, passed lateral to the bladder neck and through the anterior vaginal wall (which is also incised). A non-absorbable suture (e.g. polypropylene) is used to suspend the paraurethral tissue from the anterior rectus sheath. 'Cheese wiring' of the sutures is a problem and the long-term success rate is lower than for retropubic procedures.

Stamey procedure (Fig. 6.2) A cystoscope may be used to ensure that the suture is not placed through the bladder or urethra.

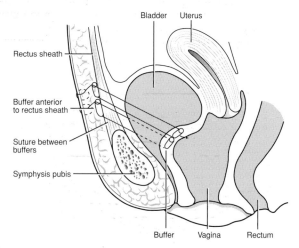

Fig. 6.2 The Stamey procedure.

Sling procedures

These are carried out using a combined abdominal and vaginal approach (Fig. 6.3). Two strips of material (e.g. abdominal rectus fascia, Mersilene, porcine dermis) are placed and sutured under the bladder neck and anchored above on both sides to either the abdominal rectus fascia or Cooper's ligaments. Although success rates are high, infection and postoperative retention may occur. The best indication is significant GSI and prolapse (e.g. large prolapse ± uterine descent ± rectocele).

Transvaginal procedures

Urethropexy (anterior colporrhaphy) See page 222. This may be indicated for large anterior vaginal wall prolapse. The success rate is significantly lower than with the retropubic procedures (40–70%), and it is usually therefore not a first-line procedure unless there are other surgical or medical risk factors to a more extensive suprapubic procedure.

Periurethral bulk enhancing agents

A number of substances (most recently microparticulate silicone, Macroplastique) have been used to inject the bladder neck to produce relative outflow obstruction. Although Macroplastique seems to be free of the disseminating complications of previous agents, reinjection is not infrequently required (Br J Urol 1995:156).

Postoperative management

Postoperatively there may be delay in voiding because of bladder-neck elevation. There are numerous regimens to prevent overdistension (>500 ml), but the simplest is to insert a suprapubic catheter at operation and allow initial free drainage. The catheter can then be clamped (e.g. on days 3–4) using a 3-hourly residual regime (the patient is asked to void as she wishes

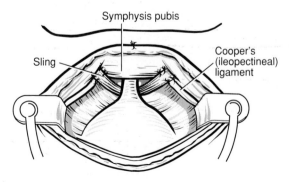

Fig. 6.3 The sling procedure.

and a postmicturition residual urine sample checked after 3 hours). Once good urine volumes are being passed (e.g. 100–200 ml) and the residuals are reducing (e.g. <150 ml) the interval between residual measurements is increased to 4–5 hours and the catheter clamped overnight. The morning residual is then checked. When residuals are all low (e.g. <150 ml), the catheter is removed. Continued difficulty in voiding after colposuspension is often caused by a degree of obstruction, and is best managed using urethral dilatation with an Otis urethrotome under urological supervision.

If overdistension occurs, the catheter should be left on free drainage for 24–48 hours. Bethanechol chloride (Myotonine) 10–20 mg PO TID or QID may improve detrusor contractility. This drug may be useful when there is a delay in re-establishing normal voiding (which may occasionally take weeks or months).

URGE SYNDROME

> The detrusor muscle contracts (either spontaneously or in response to a stimulus) while the individual is attempting to inhibit micturition. DI is a blanket term for all forms of uninhibited detrusor contractions.

Causes

- Extrinsic causes: habit, diabetes, large fluid intake, diuretics and pelvic mass (including pregnancy).
- Motor urgency: idiopathic DI and detrusor hyperreflexia (i.e. associated neuropathy).
- Sensory urgency: UTI, calculi, neoplasm, cystitis, diverticulum and atrophic changes.

Management

Urinalysis and MSU are essential. Cystourethroscopy may be of value in excluding causes of sensory urgency. DI is often chronic and can be difficult to treat.

Explanation Those with mild symptoms may need no more than this, together with advice on avoiding tea, coffee and alcohol.

Behaviour therapy (bladder drill) This aims to mimic the learning process of childhood, when conscious inhibition of the voiding reflex is acquired. Inpatient therapy involves gradually increasing the time between voiding until better control is attained, and high success rates have been achieved. This can also be carried out at home by the patient, and the use of distraction techniques can be very helpful. The self-help book *Overcome Incontinence*, by Richard Millard (Thorsons Health Series, tel. 0141 772 2281) may be helpful here.

Drugs

- Oxybutynin (e.g. Ditropan), a musculotropic relaxant and mild anticholinergic, is started at 2.5 mg OD, increased in 7 days to 2.5 mg BD and again 7 days later to 2.5 mg TID (unless the side-effects of dry mouth and blurred vision are excessive). The maximum tolerated dose is preferred (usually <10 mg/day and not greater than 15–20 mg/day). Caution is required with hepatic or renal impairment, and anticholinergics should never be used with closed-angle glaucoma or severe ulcerative colitis.
- Tolterodine (Detrusitol) 2 mg BD has a better side-effect profile than oxybutynin.
- Imipramine (a tricyclic with anticholinergic side-effects) can be used at a dose of 25–50 mg PO nocte. Being a sedative, it may have more of a role in whom nocturia is a problem.
- Desmopressin (DDAVP) 20–40 µg nocte by nasal spray (1 puff = 10 µg) significantly reduces urine production and may be used for severe nocturia (also available orally at 200 µg nocte, increasing to 400 µg if required). It has a UK licence for children, and for adults with multiple sclerosis. It has been shown to be safe in long-term use, but is contraindicated in those with cardiac insufficiency, hypertension and epilepsy. Avoid excessive fluid intake.
- HRT may be of benefit if there are significant postmenopausal atrophic changes.

Biofeedback, hypnotherapy and acupuncture These are time consuming and have lower success rates.

Surgery

- A 'Clam' ileocystoplasty is a major undertaking and is for intractable DI only. A segment of ileum on a vascular pedicle is mobilized, opened longitudinally and sutured into the bladder vault to create a reservoir. The remaining ileum is re-anastomosed. Success rates of up to 90% have been reported, but the patient will be obliged to undertake regular intermittent self-catheterization and there are problems from mucus within the bladder. Long-term follow-up is required because of the risk of adenocarcinoma in the ileal segment.
- An ileal conduit and urostomy is an option for intractable cases.

FISTULAE

> Fistulae are often complex, multiple and are usually secondary to other causes. A pathological diagnosis is very important:
>
> ● malignancy (genital, GI, GU, metastatic or postirradiation), ● trauma (particularly surgery), ● inflammation (IBD, diverticular disease, actinomycoses (e.g. with an IUCD), topical genital infections), ● obstetric problems (necrosis and lacerations), generally only third world.

History

The history is usually of uncontrolled urinary and/or faecal leakage. Urinary leakage may be intermittent (e.g. only when the bladder is full) and, in the case of a uterovesical fistula, there may be cyclical haematuria. If there is an uncertain history of urinary leakage, it is useful to place a swab high in the vagina and fill the bladder with dye (e.g. methylene blue in normal saline) through a urethral catheter. The patient is asked to mobilize and the pad inspected later for evidence of the dye. Otherwise EUA is the usual initial investigation, probing areas of granulation tissue gently to identify connections with bladder or bowel. Cystoscopy or sigmoidoscopy may confirm continuity of the probe outside the vagina. Imaging with colpography (catheter balloon in the vagina), fistulography, cystography, hysteroscopy, IVU and small bowel radiographs may also be helpful.

Management principles

- If the fistula occurs in the immediate postoperative period, consider arranging immediate closure.
- Closure of later postoperative fistulae should be delayed for 2–3 months to allow inflammation to settle.
- If there is malignancy, treat and consider diversion or exenteration.
- If there is IBD, treat medically before closure of the fistula.
- Do not close a urinary fistula if there is no residual sphincter, as this simply leads to incontinence from the urethra.
- Any urinary calculi must be removed before surgery.
- General health is important. Correct anaemia.

Surgical options

These should only be undertaken by someone with a subspecialist interest. Options include conservative management, laying open (e.g. for a low anal lesion in IBD), transvaginal closure in layers (e.g. for midvaginal fistulae), saucerization (closure with a purse-string suture if there is little extra tissue), or via the transabdominal route (using a transvesical or transperitoneal approach ±grafting). Ureteric fistulae may require construction using a Boari flap, or a loop of bowel, or re-anastomosis to the contralateral ureter,

GYNAECOLOGICAL ONCOLOGY

> All gynaecological cancers should be managed by a multidisciplinary team comprising a specialist gynaecologist, clinical/medical oncology and palliative medicine specialist. Where possible, patients should be entered into trials.

BENIGN AND PREMALIGNANT DISEASE OF THE VULVA

Pruritus vulvae

This is commoner in those aged >40 years and may be caused by infection (candida, pediculosis, threadworms), eczema, dermatitis (consider patch testing), lichen sclerosis, lichen planus, VIN, vulval carcinoma, diabetes mellitus, uraemia, liver failure or irritation from a vaginal discharge. A biopsy may be necessary. If no cause is found, avoid irritants and bathwater additives, use soap substitutes, dry gently (e.g. with a hairdryer), wear loose cotton clothing and avoid nylon tights. Hydrocortisone cream 2.5% BD for 3 weeks followed by hydrocortisone cream 1% daily as maintenance is useful, as is the use of soap substitutes (e.g. oilatum). Antihistamines (e.g. terfenadine 60 mg BD) may also be of help. Primary or secondary depression may also warrant treatment.

Vulvodynia

This is chronic vulvar discomfort, especially that characterized by the complaint of pruritus, burning, stinging, irritation or rawness. No one factor can be identified as the specific cause, and indeed there appear to be clinically definable differences between groups of patients. It may occasionally be associated with previous sexual abuse. Vulvar vestibulitis is a chronic clinical syndrome, with erythema, severe pain on entry or to vestibular touch, and tenderness to pressure localized within the vestibule. If symptoms have been present less than 3 months there is often response to topical corticosteroids. If chronic, treatment is empirical and symptomatic, with vestibular resection being considered only as a last resort. Essential vulvodynia refers to the description of constant, unremitting burning localized to the vulva which may respond to low-dose tricyclic antidepressants (e.g. amitriptyline 10 mg nocte increasing to 50 mg). Vestibular papillomatosis is used to describe the presence of multiple papillae that may cover the surface of the labia minora, and is likely to be an asymptomatic variant of normal. The Vulvar Pain Society is a self-help group for patients with vulvodynia (PO Box 20, Worsley, UK).

Ulcers

Ulcers may be:

- Aphthous (yellow base).

- Herpetic (exquisitely painful multiple ulceration, see p. 191).
- Syphilitic (indurated and painless, see p. 192).
- Associated with Crohn's disease ('like knife cuts in skin').
- A feature of Behçet's disease. (This is a chronic painful condition with aphthous, genital and ocular ulceration. Treatment is difficult; the COC or topical steroids may be tried.)
- Malignant.
- Associated with lichen planus or Stevens–Johnson syndrome.
- Tropical (lymphogranuloma venereum, chancroid, granuloma inguinale).

ISSVD classification for benign vulval diseases

Lichen sclerosis This can present at any age, but is more common in the older patient and usually presents with pruritus, and less commonly with dyspareunia or pain. The skin appears white, thin and crinkly, but may be thickened and keratotic if there is coexistent squamous cell hyperplasia. There may also be clitoral or labial adhesions. Diagnosis is by biopsy and there is an association with autoimmune disorders (PA, thyroid disease, IDDM, SLE, primary biliary cirrhosis or bullous pemphygoid) in <10%. It is non-neoplastic but may coexist with VIN and there is an association with subsequent development of squamous cell carcinoma of the vulva (probably in 2–9%). Long-term 6- to 12-monthly follow-up is probably warranted. Treat only if symptomatic (e.g. Dermovate BD initially, reducing gradually to hydrocortisone 1% BD, OD or less as symptoms require. Eosin paint 2% may also be of help. Vulvectomy has no role, the recurrence being ≈50%.

Squamous cell hyperplasia This frequently presents in premenopausal women with severe pruritus. Diagnosis is again by biopsy and treatment is with hydrocortisone, as for lichen sclerosis.

Other dermatoses These include:

- *Allergic/irritant dermatosis* This may be caused by detergents, perfume, condom lubricants, chlorine in swimming pools or podophyllin paint. There may be secondary infection. Remove the irritant and treat with emollients ± topical corticosteroids.
- *Psoriasis* The vulva is an unusual site for this, but if present moderately potent steroids are better than coal tar.
- *Intertrigo with candida* This responds to antifungal preparations.
- *Lichen planus* This appears as purple-white papules with a shiny surface and keratinized area and may respond to strong steroids ± azathioprine or PUVA. It is usually idiopathic, but can be drug related, and tends to resolve within 2 years. Surgery should be avoided.

Varieties of intraepithelial neoplasia
These neoplasias involve neoplastic cells within the confines of the epithelium.

Squamous VIN This is classified as class 1, 2 or 3, depending on the severity (the names 'Bowen's disease' and 'Bowenoid papulosis' have been used to describe atypical squamous lesions, but are part of the same process of VIN). It is considered that HPV may be important in the aetiology. Many cases are asymptomatic, although pruritus is present in one- to two-thirds and pain is an occasional feature. Lesions may be papular and rough surfaced, resembling warts, or macular with indistinct borders. White lesions represent hyperkeratosis and pigmentation is common. The lesions tend to be multifocal in women under 40 years and unifocal in the postmenopausal age group. Diagnosis is by biopsy which may be taken at colposcopy, either with LA or under GA. As the natural history is so uncertain, treatment is controversial. Regression has been observed (particularly low-grade VIN), but progression of high-grade VIN to invasion may occur in approximately 6% of cases and up to 15% of those with VIN 3 may have superficial invading vulval cancer. Treatment of VIN may be indicated in those >45 years, those who are immunosuppressed and those with multifocal lower genital tract neoplasia. The main treatment is wide local excision (the exception is VIN 3 on the clitoris in young women – use a Nd-YAG laser). Use a colposcope to inspect the vulva (keratinization may make visualization of abnormal cells difficult) and then take a biopsy with a 4 mm trephine under LA or GA. Apply Monsel's solution to the base (you must also check perianal area, as there may be AIN).

Melanoma in situ This is uncommon.

Non-squamous VIN (Paget's disease) This is also uncommon. There is a poorly demarcated, often multifocal, eczematoid lesion which is associated in 25% with adenocarcinoma either in the pelvis or at a distant site. Treatment is by wide local excision.

VULVAL CARCINOMA

Eighty per cent occur in those aged >65 years. Presentation is with pruritus vulvae (70%), mass or ulcer (57%), or bleeding (25%). Two-thirds of squamous tumours occur on the labia majora (especially anteriorly). The rest occur on the clitoris, labia minora, posterior fourchette and perineum. Spread is by *embolization* to the superficial inguinal, deep inguinal and external iliac nodes. Diagnosis is with EUA and excision biopsy, although outpatient biopsy may be appropriate (FNA of groin nodes has a 90% sensitivity and excellent specificity if a node is palpable). USS, CT scanning and lymphangiography have little role in assessing groin nodes. It is also important to examine the cervix and check a cervical smear as there may be co-existing CIN or a cervical carcinoma.

Pathology of malignant vulval tumours

- 85% are squamous;
- 5% are malignant melanomas;
- the rest are Bartholin's tumours, basal cell tumours or adenocarcinoma;
- verrucous carcinoma is rare.

Surgical treatment

The staging of vulval carcinomas is given in Table 7.1.

TABLE 7.1   FIGO staging of vulval carcinoma

Stage	Definition
I$_A$	Tumour less than 2.0 cm in dimension and less than 1 mm of stromal invasion. No lymph vascular space invasion and no nodal disease
I$_B$	Tumour less than 2.0 cm in dimension but with more than 1 mm of stromal invasion
II	Tumour of more than 2.0 cm dimension confined to the vulva or perineum with negative nodes
III	Tumour of any size with spread to lower urethra, ± vagina, ± anus, ± unilateral groin lymph node metastases
IV$_A$	Tumour invades any of the following: upper urethra, bladder mucosa, rectal mucosa, pelvic bone ± bilateral groin nodes
IV$_B$	Any distant metastases, including pelvic nodes

Generally the 5 year survival is said to be 80% if the groin nodes are negative and 40% if they are positive, i.e. the most important predictor of survival is regional nodal disease. Factors predictive of nodal disease are: clinically suspicious groin nodes, grade of tumour (well differentiated vs poorly differentiated), age of patient (old vs young) and presence of lymphatic or vascular space invasion. Depth of stromal invasion is particularly related to groin node involvement:

- <1 mm invasion, no positive groin nodes;
- <3 mm invasion, 12% positive groin nodes;
- <5 mm invasion, 16% positive groin nodes.

Treatment is wide local excision for I$_A$ tumours (i.e. excision which includes a 10 mm margin of normal tissue both laterally and deep to the tumour). For lateralized stage I$_B$/II disease (i.e. a lesion where the medial surgical excision line will clear a midline structure (e.g. clitoris, anus, urethra, vagina) by a minimum margin of 10 mm) wide local excision + ipsilateral groin node dissection is carried out. Contralateral groin node exploration is only carried out if the ipsilateral nodes are positive (if the ipsilateral groin nodes are negative the risk of contralateral nodes being positive is <1%). In centralized I$_B$/II disease, wide local excision and bilateral groin dissections are appropriate, i.e. there is a move away from radical vulvectomy because of its mutilating nature. Radical vulvectomy would still be appropriate for an elderly woman with VIN affecting the entire vulval epithelium who has also developed vulval cancer. Groin explorations are carried out through separate incisions, and the wound should be drained for around 7–10 days under suction, as lymph fluid accumulates and breakdown is common.

Further treatment

If more than two groin nodes are positive (microscopic involvement) or one is involved (macroscopic) there is a 15–20% chance of pelvic node involvement and adjuvant radiotherapy is probably appropriate. If disease is advanced (i.e. grossly involved nodes) the options are chemotherapy and radiotherapy followed by surgery, or, if there is functional impairment, radical excision (e.g. colostomy, urinary diversion with loop conduit).

Recurrence

Recurrence of the excised tumour at the primary site is unusual providing a 10 mm margin has been achieved. The epithelium is likely to be unstable, however, and new vulval tumours may arise. Treatment of recurrence is surgical, although interstitial radiotherapy may be appropriate. Look for signs of tumour spread to nodes.

OTHER TUMOURS

Malignant melanoma This is histologically assessed in terms of depth of invasion (the Breslow thickness). If invasion is <1 mm the prognosis is good, otherwise it is bleak. Wide local excision is carried out (one-third have lymph node spread at presentation). Chemotherapy and radiotherapy are of little use.

Bartholin's gland tumours These may be squamous, transitional cell or adenocarcinomas. Treatment is by radical excision to include the ischiorectal fossa.

Basal cell carcinoma This is treated by wide local excision.

Verrucous carcinoma This is a variant of squamous cell carcinoma, but is slow growing and rarely metastasizes. Treatment is by wide local excision but without groin node exploration. Radiotherapy may transform it to an anaplastic form *and has no role*.

CERVICAL SMEARS

The cervical smear programme allows screening for dyskaryosis (abnormality of individual cells with hyperchromasia, irregular nuclei and multinucleation). This is classified as mild, moderate or severe and suggests the need for colposcopy ± biopsy. Biopsy identifies the histological diagnosis of dysplasia (abnormality of arrangement of cells), which is also classified as mild, moderate or severe (CIN I, II and III) depending on whether the atypical cells are confined to the basal layers or extend to the epithelial surface. Screening is undertaken every 3 years from the age of 20 years to 60 years, although there is evidence to suggest that it may be discontinued at the age of 50 in those with a normal smear history. There is a 10–15% incidence of false-positive and false-negative smear results.

[handwritten margin notes: 20 6, 64 ; sensitivity 0.52, specificity 0.94]

Screening is based on the assumption that CIN is a progressive disorder, but in reality it may revert to normal. The risk of CIN III progressing to invasive disease is uncertain, but estimates from studies range from 14% to 70%, and is likely to be around the lower end of this estimate. Cervical smears are also used as follow-up after colposcopy and vault smears *may* be used as follow-up after treatment for cervical cancer. There are *regional variations* in smear reporting and management. An example of the management depending on smear results is shown in Table 7.2.

TABLE 7.2 Cervical cytology, associated pathology and subsequent management

Smear	Risk of having CIN II or III on biopsy	Management	If next smear(s) negative
Normal	0.1%	Repeat in 3 years if no previous abnormality	Routine recall
Inflammatory	<6%	Repeat in 3 years if no previous abnormality	Routine recall
Borderline	20–37%	Repeat in 6 months	Repeat in 1 year, then 2 years, then routine recall. Colposcopy if 3 borderline smears
Mild dyskaryosis	30–50% (note that 30% have CIN I, 30–60% regress and 10% may progress to CIN III)	Repeat in 3 months	Repeat in 1 year, then 2 years, then routine recall. Colposcopy if 2 mildly dyskaryotic smears
Moderate dyskaryosis	50–70%	Colposcopy	Repeat at follow-up
Severe dyskaryosis	80–90%	Colposcopy	Repeat at follow-up
Invasion suspected	50% have invasion	Urgent colposcopy	

Notes

- Adenocarcinoma of the cervix may also be detected on cervical smears, although colposcopy only identifies ≈50% of endocervical adenocarcinomas. The vast majority are diagnosed by large loop excision. If there are abnormal glandular cells on the smear, arrange a pelvic scan to look at the ovaries and tubes, transvaginal scan (±hysteroscopy) to look at the endometrium, and colposcopy and LLETZ to look at the endocervical canal.
- Koilocytosis suggests papilloma virus infection, often the more benign subtypes (e.g. types 6–11). These can co-exist with other subtypes.
- Other possible infections identified include HSV, *Trichomonas vaginalis*, *Candida albicans* and gardnerella species (see p. 189).

Future developments

HPV subtypes 16 and 18 have been detected in 50–80% of woman with CIN 2 and CIN 3 and in 90% of invasive squamous cervical cancers. It may therefore be useful to increase cytological surveillance in those found to have these subtypes, or to use their detection to determine treatment for those with mildly dyskaryotic smears. The acquisition of HPV infection in most women, however, is transient, and further research is required in this area before such surveillance becomes a useful tool.

COLPOSCOPY

Cervix

> The transformation zone is a circumferential region of tissue between the vaginal (squamous) and the endocervical (columnar) epithelium. It is composed of columnar epithelium which has descended onto the ectocervix, and it metaplases to a varying degree to squamous epithelium. This process exposes it to neoplastic transformation.

History and investigation

Take a history and insert a speculum, looking for condylomata, leukoplakia (hyperkeratinization which may conceal an invasive lesion) and invasive disease itself ± tumour, ulceration or atypical vessels.

   Apply 3% acetic acid. This coagulates protein and stains abnormal cells (which have a more rapid turnover and therefore more protein) white:

- Columnar epithelium blanches white briefly and has a villous or furrowed surface.
- Squamous metaplasia appears glassy white but can be hard to differentiate from CIN.

- Warts show as small lesions with looped capillaries ± satellite lesions.
- CIN: there are clearly defined margins enclosing a mosaic vascular pattern with patches of acetowhite separated by red vessels (punctation represents vessels seen 'end on'). The intervessel distance increases with more severe lesions, and bizarre branching with coarse punctation and atypical vessels suggests invasive disease.

   Lugol's iodine (Schiller's test) stains glycogen (in normal cells) mahogany brown. Non-staining areas are termed Schiller's negative.

Management

If the transformation zone is seen and there is no abnormality, return to the routine smear programme (although excision may be warranted in a grossly abnormal smear). If an abnormality is seen, infiltrate the paracervical tissue on either side of the cervix with 5 ml of Citanest and Octapressin for loop diathermy excision (which acts as biopsy and treatment). Biopsy followed by local destruction is a more conservative alternative option for those subsequently shown to have no more than CIN 1.

Notes

- The squamocolumnar junction is marked by the lower limit of normal columnar epithelium, not the upper limit of squamous epithelium.
- If the transformation zone is not seen, a deep cervical loop diathermy excision is appropriate.
- Local treatment for CIN 1 should not be carried out before a specimen has been taken for histology and never for suspected invasive disease or AIS. If smear is severely dyskaryotic and obvious acetowhite, LLETZ may be appropriate. Cone biopsy by scalpel is rarely used, as there is a significantly greater morbidity than with LLETZ or biopsy.
- Suspected AIS should be biopsied, as normal colposcopy does not exclude abnormal glandular cells.
- In a previously treated cervix, excision is preferable to ablation.
- Hysterectomy may be appropriate for a patient with CIN 3 who has completed her family and who wishes assurance of cure and/or would be difficult to follow-up.

   A biopsy may demonstrate adenocarcinoma in situ which is classified as low or high grade. The natural history of this is not known (i.e. if low-grade disease leads to high-grade disease), but it is known that high-grade disease may progress to invasive cancer. Consider simple hysterectomy for high-grade disease if the patient's family is complete. Otherwise, a deep cervical cone (usually this means a knife cone biopsy) is required. If the margins are negative, arrange an annual smear and colposcopy. If the margins are positive, recommend simple hysterectomy (50% of women will have residual adenocarcinoma in situ and up to 10% may have microinvasive adenocarcinoma).

5% of pts. treated for CIN will have recurrent dis. ē in 2 yrs. Although no. of recurrence is small. Long term f/u is still reqd.

Vagina

Vaginal intraepithelial neoplasia (VAIN) is rare (as is vaginal cancer) and again the natural history unknown (i.e. if VAIN 1 leads to VAIN 2, and to VAIN 3, or if the different classes of VAIN arise de novo). Thirty per cent of VAIN 3 develops into invasive disease. Ninety per cent of VAIN 3 is in the upper vagina and in 60% of these cases it is confluent with CIN 3. It is appropriate to carry out a hysterectomy for CIN 3, providing the patient's family is complete, with a good cuff of vagina (to avoid VAIN in the 'dog ears' at the vault).

Vulva

(See Vulval Intraepithelial Neoplasia, p. 237.)

CERVICAL CANCER

> Clinical presentation is with intermenstrual bleeding, postcoital bleeding or following abnormal cytology. Spread is to the internal and external iliac, obturator and common iliac nodes, then to the para-aortic nodes. Tumour also spreads locally to involve the bladder, ureters, rectum and bone. Blood-borne metastases spread to liver, lungs and bone occur.

Pathology

- 80% of tumours are squamous. There is an increased incidence with early age at first intercourse, number of partners, smoking, immunocompromise, a previous partner of a woman with cervical cancer and the presence of human papilloma virus serotypes 16 and 18.
- 20% are adenocarcinomas.
- Adenosquamous has a worse prognosis than squamous cancer.
- Malignant melanomas and sarcomas are rare.

Staging (see Table 7.3)

This is *clinical*, based on EUA, speculum and rectovaginal examination (? parametrial involvement), cystoscopy, curettage and biopsy ±IVU. Although additional investigations do not form part of the staging process, there is increasing use of MRI or CT scan to assess the size of the tumour and the presence of nodal metastases. If nodes are radiologically suspicious and the cervical lesion is <4 cm in diameter it may be more appropriate to avoid surgery and treat with chemo- and radiotherapy. This also applies when the tumour is more than 4.0 cm in dimension, even if still confined to the cervix (as these have often metastasized to pelvic nodes).

TABLE 7.3   FIGO staging of cervical cancer

Stage	Invasion	Pelvic nodes	Para-aortic nodes	Prognosis (5 year survival)	Treatment
IA1	Depth of invasion up to 3 mm and width up to 7 mm (includes early stromal invasion of up to 1 mm)	<1%		84–90% if tumour diameter <3 cm; 85% will have negative pelvic nodes and 95% of these patients should remain disease free	Local excision; if margins of a cone clear (i.e. no residual tumour or CIN) then conization is adequate, with no need for pelvic lymphadenectomy
IA2	Depth of invasion between 3 and 5 mm (i.e. 3.1–5 mm) and width up to 7 mm	6.5%	≈0%		Simple hysterectomy and pelvic lymphadenectomy
IB1	Tumour confined to the cervix and diameter less than 4 cm			66% if tumour >3 cm	Radical hysterectomy and pelvic lymphadenectomy
IB2	Tumour confined to the cervix and diameter more than 4 cm	15%	5%		Radiotherapy and chemotherapy
IIA	Upper two-thirds of vagina	25%	15%	62%	
IIB	Upper two-thirds of vagina plus parametrial disease				
IIIA	Lower third of vagina				
IIIB	Pelvic side wall ± hydronephrosis	35%	25%	40%	
IVA	Bladder, rectum	50%	40%	15%	
IVB	Beyond pelvis				

Notes

- It remains unclear whether in 1A2 disease the presence of lymphatic or vascular space involvement increases the risk of pelvic nodal disease. This is also controversial in 1A1 disease, and those who believe it is would advocate pelvic node sampling for 1A1 disease with lymphatic or vascular space involvement.
- If pelvic nodes are positive, up to 60% of patients have positive para-aortic nodes.

Management

For small tumours, radiotherapy is as effective as surgery, but surgery causes less long-term morbidity. Ovaries should be conserved in young women.

Radical hysterectomy and bilateral pelvic lymphadenectomy This carries an operative mortality <1% with a subsequent risk of infection, PTE, haemorrhage, vesicovaginal and uterovaginal fistulae. There are medium-term problems with reduced bladder sensation and voiding difficulties, together with long-term problems of high residual volumes, recurrent UTIs and stress incontinence.

Radiotherapy Generally patients receive radical pelvic radiotherapy with external beam X-ray treatment (telotherapy) to the pelvis. Before it is given it is important to ensure that there are no distant metastases. The patient attends a simulator room for planning of treatment, which is then given in 20 fractions over 4 weeks. It can be given as parallel opposed fields or anterior and posterior fields. Generally, if the tumour is large and growing into the sacral hollow, anteroposterior fields are used. If there is a large exophytic bleeding tumour telotherapy causes tumour shrinkage and stops the bleeding. Diarrhoea and urinary urgency/frequency occur during the treatment as well as marked tiredness. After this patients usually attend for an EUA and insertion of a vaginal delivery system (for brachytherapy). Delivery is by selectron machine usually with a caudal block in a room with lead shields. The patient is awake during the treatment which takes 12–18 hours and many patients get a second insertion 2–3 weeks after the first.

In the pelvic node positive patient after surgery, adjuvant radiotherapy has not been shown to significantly impact on survival but does decrease pelvic recurrence (relapse is confined to the pelvis in only 40%). Most centres give adjuvant pelvic X-ray treatment if there is more than one microscopic node involved or one positive macroscopic node.

Treat acute diarrhoea with low residue diet and imodium. There are long-term problems in 5–10% of cases: chronic diarrhoea from small bowel damage (beginning on average after 10 months), radiation cystitis (beginning on average after 22 months) and PR bleeding (peak incidence at 2 years). Vaginal stenosis causes sexual dysfunction (encourage the use of vaginal dilators). Radiation to para-aortic nodes carries significant mortality and chemotherapy is more appropriate.

Recurrence:
- After surgery: give radiotherapy ± chemotherapy.
- After radiotherapy: if the recurrence is small and central with no evidence of nodal spread, consider anterior, posterior or complete pelvic exenteration with urinary and/or bowel diversion ± vaginal and pelvic floor reconstruction. The operative mortality is 10–20% and there is major morbidity. The 5 year survival is ≈30%.

ENDOMETRIAL CARCINOMA

> The majority (80%) of endometrial carcinomas occur postmenopausally; it is rare before the age of 35 years. Risk factors include low parity, late menopause, obesity, PCOS, unopposed oestrogen preparations and diabetes mellitus. Use of the COC reduces the risk. Presentation is usually with abnormal bleeding. Fifty per cent of postmenopausal discharges with a pyometra have carcinoma.

Pathology

Adenocarcinoma is by far the commonest and may be:

- endometrioid;
- adenocarcinoma with squamous metaplasia (adenoacanthoma), which is slightly less aggressive;
- adenosquamous, papillary serous and clear cell tumours, which carry a poorer prognosis.

Soft tissue sarcomas are rare, but usually arise from the uterus (although they can be from an ovary, fallopian tube, the cervix, vulva or vagina):

- 60% mixed Mullerian tumours (MMT), the classification depending on whether malignancy is in the epithelial component, stromal or both;
- 28% leiomyosarcoma;
- 8% endometrial stromal carcinoma (can be low or high grade);
- 4% others.

Surgical treatment

Staging The staging is *surgical* (Table 7.4). After diagnosis by biopsy ± hysteroscopy ± TVS, assess further with U&E, LFTs and CXR ± CT or MRI. Consider bowel preparation only if surgical difficulty is anticipated with the bowel. At laparotomy take peritoneal washings with saline and examine for pelvic and para-aortic nodes as well as omental and liver spread.

A TAH and BSO should be carried out, but the role of pelvic or para-aortic lymph node sampling is controversial. It may be possible to avoid unnecessary postoperative X-ray treatment if the pelvic nodes are negative. The MRC ASTEC trial is currently looking at the role of pelvic lymphadenectomy in the 'high risk' clinical stage 1 disease (i.e. clear cell, papillary serous or adenosquamous pathology, grade 3 endometrioid carcinoma or any case where myoinvasion is suspected to be >50%).

If there is spread into the abdomen, debulking is advised.

TABLE 7.4   FIGO staging of endometrial carcinoma

Stage	Definition	Pelvic node involvement	5 year survival
Iᴀ	Tumour limited to the endometrium		
Iʙ	Growth that has invaded <50% of myometrial thickness	<20%	70%
Iᴄ	Growth that has invaded >50% of myometrial thickness		
IIᴀ	Endocervical glandular involvement only	20%	56%
IIʙ	Cervical stromal involvement		
IIIᴀ	Invades seroserosal surface of uterus, ± adnexa, ± positive washings		
IIIʙ	Vaginal metastases	35%	30%
IIIᴄ	Metastases to pelvic or para-aortic nodes		
IVᴀ	Tumour invasion of bladder ± bowel		
IVʙ	Distant metastases including intra-abdominal ± inguinal lymph nodes	50%	20%

Postoperative management There is no evidence that adjuvant pelvic radiotherapy increases survival, but it does reduce the risk of pelvic relapse

● If grade 1 and Iᴀ or Iʙ, then no further treatment is required.
● If grade 2 and Iᴀ or Iʙ, consider vault irradiation.
● If grade 3, or >Iʙ, or adenosquamous, clear cell or papillary serous, use adjuvant pelvic radiotherapy. Those with a papillary serous carcinoma may be given chemotherapy.

In addition to staging, prognosis is also dependent on age (younger better), grade and ploidy (euploidy better).

Recurrence Most relapses occur early (i.e. within 2 years of primary treatment). This is commonest in the vaginal vault, lungs, bone, vagina, liver, inguinal and supraclavicular nodes.

● If the patient is not receiving radiotherapy, refer to radiotherapist.
● If there is late central pelvic recurrence in the irradiated patient, consider exenteration (see p. 246).
● 15–20% may respond to high-dose progesterone (e.g. Provera 30–100 mg TID).
● Single-agent chemotherapy (e.g. cisplatinum) may also be appropriate.

FALLOPIAN TUBE TUMOURS

These are very rare. They are usually serous carcinomas and tend to occur postmenopausally, are unilateral and classically present with postmenopausal bleeding, a watery discharge and abdominal pain. Commonly, however, presentation is similar to ovarian carcinoma. Spread, staging and prognosis are also as for ovarian carcinoma.

OVARIAN CARCINOMA

The peak incidence in the age range 50–70 years and carcinoma is more likely with nulliparity and those with a positive family history. The use of the COC is protective. Presentation is usually with abdominal pain and swelling, but may be with urinary frequency, weight loss, dyspeptic symptoms or abnormal menses. Three-quarters of cases have spread outside the pelvis at presentation (to the peritoneum, diaphragm, para-aortic lymph nodes, liver and lung) hence the overall 5 year survival of 29%. Epithelial tumours account for 80% of all ovarian neoplasms and 90% of all primary malignant ovarian tumours.

Pathology of ovarian tumours

Epithelial tumours

Serous tumours

- Adenoma cystadenoma, papillary cystadenoma or cystadenofibroma: these are often uni- or bilocular.
- Adenocarcinoma: these tend to be large, partially cystic and partially solid.

Mucinous tumours

- Cystadenoma: these are multilocular. Rupture may lead to pseudomyxoma peritonei (may lead to death from small bowel obstruction and cachexia).
- Cystadenocarcinoma: these are often largely solid and may also lead to pseudomyxoma peritonei.

Endometrioid tumours These are rare. Differentiate from secondary endometrial carcinoma.

Brenner tumours These are composed of fibrous elements and transitional epithelium from Wolffian remnants. They are usually benign but, if malignant, a bladder tumour must be excluded.

Clear cell tumours These are Mullerian in origin and are usually highly malignant. They are bilateral in 10%, and in 15% of cases are associated with an endometrial primary tumour as well.

Borderline tumours These are a separate entity and are defined as carcinomata of low malignant potential lacking stromal invasion, but may have apparent extraovarian spread. Indeed in ≈20% of cases there are 'metastases' at diagnosis. The tumours are largely serous (50% bilateral) or mucinous (5% bilateral) and carry an excellent prognosis (e.g. 5 year survival: stage I, 97%; stage III, 85%). Nonetheless, ≈50% will eventually die from the disease.

Sex cord/stromal tumours

Granulosa cell tumours

- Adult: these usually occur at age ≥60 years, but can occur prepubertally and are solid. Three-quarters have endocrine function (PMB, irregular cycle, precocious pseudopuberty). They tend to recur late, and monitoring with G125 and oestradiol is sometimes appropriate. There is 50% survival at 20 years (prognosis is poor if there is extraovarian spread at diagnosis).
- Juvenile: these are usually unilateral and large. Only 5% are malignant, but those that are are aggressive and are treated with chemotherapy.

Thecoma These are solid, yellow, usually postmenopausal and almost always benign.

Androblastoma (arrhenoblastoma)

- Sertoli: these are 70% oestrogenic, 20% androgenic and 10% no secretion. They are usually benign.
- Leydig cell: these are very rare.
- Mixed Sertoli/Leydig: these are also very rare.

Germ cell tumours

These are the commonest tumours in the <30 year old age group, but overall are more common in those aged >40 years. Only 2–3% are malignant (although ≈30% are malignant in those <20 years old). They are categorized according to the degree of cellular differentiation.

No differentiation

- Dysgerminoma (a completely undifferentiated tumour): this accounts for 50% of malignant germ cell tumours and usually presents in the <30 year old age group. The tumours are very radio- and chemosensitive, but are treated with chemotherapy to preserve ovarian function. In 10–15% of cases there is bilateral disease.

Extraembryonic differentiation

- Malignant ovarian choriocarcinoma: these secrete hCG and may present with precocious pseudopuberty. They have a poor prognosis and do not respond well to chemotherapy (unlike uterine trophoblastic disease).
- Yolk sac tumours (endodermal sinus tumours): these occur in the age group 14–20 years and secrete αFP. They usually occur unilaterally and are chemosensitive.

Embryonic

- Mature cyst (dermoid): in 90% of cases these are in women of reproductive age. Overall, 10% are bilateral. They are usually unilocular, often with a focal hillock, squamous epithelium and skin appendages. There is a focus of malignant change in 1% of cases, and these carry a poor prognosis.

- Immature solid tumour: these are rare, malignant (usually squamous or neural malignant tissue) and secrete hCG and αFP.

Miscellaneous These include gonadoblastoma (benign, from streak ovary or testis), Leydig cell tumours or small cell carcinoma.

Metastases These may occur from gastric, breast and colonic tumours. A Krukenberg tumour is a metastasis from any mucus secreting adenocarcinoma. Meig syndrome may occur with a fibroma, Brenner tumour, thecoma or granulosa cell tumour.

Management

Malignancy in an ovarian cyst is more likely in those aged >45 years, or in whom cysts are bilateral, or where there are ascites, or solid areas within the cyst, or an irregular growth on the capsule, or where the cyst is fixed.

Although overall there is an increased risk of ovarian cancer in those with a family history (RR = 1.1 for mother, 3.8 for sister and 6.0 for daughter), the risk is small for most categories, except those with more than one affected relative. If one affected primary relative has ovarian cancer and it was diagnosed when she was <50 years old, the risk increases to 1:20 (5%). If there are two affected primary relatives and both develop disease under the age of 50 years there is a >50% chance of disease being hereditary. The life-long risk of a family member with this family history developing ovarian carcinoma is 25%.

Five to ten per cent of cases of ovarian carcinoma are attributable to hereditary factors, particularly the breast–ovarian cancer tumour suppressor BRCA1 and BRCA2 genes which are associated with a 10–50% lifetime risk of developing ovarian carcinoma. Mismatch repair genes, associated with cancer of the colorectum, endometrium, stomach, urinary tract and small bowel are also responsible for a small proportion of this group. BRAC1 mutations are found in ≈80% of families with histories of both ovarian and breast cancer, but overall this mutation accounts for only 2% of cases of breast cancer and 3% of cases of ovarian cancer. Those with these genes may warrant 6–12 monthly screening with Ca125 and USS. Bilateral oophorectomy after completion of the family may also be advocated, but this does not offer complete protection, probably due to 'ovarian carcinoma' arising de novo from the peritoneum.

Staging

See Table 7.5.

Investigations and treatment

Initial investigations should be with USS (±CT or MRI), U&E, LFT, Ca125 and CXR (αFP, hCG and oestradiol should also be sent if a sex-cord/stromal or germ cell tumour is suspected). Peritoneal fluid cytology may demonstrate malignant cells (but is unnecessary if laparotomy is planned anyway).

TABLE 7.5 FIGO staging of ovarian cancer

Stage	Definition	5 year survival
IA	One ovary	60–70%,
IB	Both ovaries	but can be
IC	IA or IB with ruptured capsule, tumour on the surface of the capsule, positive peritoneal washings or malignant ascites	95% for IA
IIA	Extension to uterus and tubes	
IIB	Extension to other pelvis tissues (e.g. pelvic nodes, pouch of Douglas)	30%
IIC	IIA or IIB with ruptured capsule, positive peritoneal washings or malignant ascites	
IIIA	Pelvic tumour with microscopic peritoneal spread	
IIIB	Pelvic tumour with peritoneal spread <2 cm	
IIIC	Abdominal implants >2 cm ± positive retroperitoneal or inguinal nodes	10%
IV	Liver parenchymal disease. Distant metastases. If pleural effusion, must have malignant cells	

Pleural fluid, if present, may also demonstrate malignant cells and this should be aspirated prior to surgery. Ca125 is not a specific marker and may be elevated with many intra-abdominal problems, including PID, endometriosis and after surgery itself. Preoperative bowel preparation should be given if bowel surgery is anticipated. On opening the peritoneum, aspirate peritoneal fluid or take washings with saline. Conservative surgery (with removal of one ovary) may be warranted if the patient is young, plans further family, has unilateral disease and has no ascites (alternatively, a per-operative frozen section may be used). Otherwise TAH, BSO and infracolic omentectomy should be performed. Per-operative rupture of intact cysts probably has no adverse prognostic effect providing careful peritoneal toilet is performed. If there is extensive disease, cytoreductive surgery (debulking) is appropriate to improve quality of life, improve response to chemotherapy, prolong remission and increase median survival. Some surgeons would consider pelvic and para-aortic node sampling to ensure accurate staging in apparent IA and IB cases.

Postoperative chemotherapy is usually given for epithelial tumours if the staging is >IA (or for IA if this is poorly differentiated). Germ cell tumours are very sensitive to chemotherapy, so fertility-conserving surgery in the young patient is appropriate; the majority of young patients are cured even if metastatic disease is present. Sex cord–stromal tumours may occur at either end of the age spectrum. Most are stage I at presentation and can be effectively treated with conservative surgery if young. Late recurrences occur, with variable response to chemotherapy, and further surgery may be required.

Many studies using Cisplatin based combinations have achieved 70–80% overall response rates with up to 50% complete clinical response. A few years ago the combination of Cisplatin and Cyclophosphamide with or without addition of Doxorubicin was considered standard therapy. However, the results of two large recent randomized studies have shown that treatment with Paclitaxel and Cisplatin given every 3 weeks for six cycles has an improved response rate, progression-free survival, and overall survival compared to the combination of Cisplatin and Cyclophosphamide. Median duration of survival is increased from about 2 to 3 years for advanced (>Ic) stage disease. The problem is that the regime with Paclitaxel has significant side-effects (neurological, alopecia, allergic). Studies are now attempting to see if substituting Cisplatin with Carboplatin reduces toxicity.

Screening for ovarian cancer

The poor survival rates associated with advanced ovarian cancer have contributed to the concern that effective screening tests be developed. Presently there is no evidence that screening the general population is useful or cost-effective. Women with a family history that are deemed to be at high risk should be considered for the national familial ovarian cancer screening study run through clinical genetics centres.

GESTATIONAL TROPHOBLASTIC DISEASE

> This is an abnormal proliferation of trophoblastic tissue which occurs in approximately 1.5:1000 UK pregnancies. Large reported differences in incidence between different racial groups have not been confirmed. In the UK management after ERPOC should be confined to one of the three centres: Charing Cross, London; Ninewells, Dundee; Weston Park, Sheffield (RCOG Guideline No. 18, 1999).

Pathology

Hydatidiform mole This is the commonest type of gestational trophoblastic disease.

Partial hydatidiform mole This is triploid (one set of maternal and two sets of paternal chromosomes, usually 69 XXY). There may be an abnormal conceptus in which the fetus often dies early in the first trimester. Although 1% invade (invasive mole) and a few of these develop metastases, they virtually never become choriocarcinoma. Only 0.5% require treatment after ERPOC.

Complete hydatidiform mole This is androgenetically diploid, although the female nuclear DNA is inactivated. There is duplication of one haploid sperm (XX) in 90% and the rest are dispermic (usually XY). The abnormal conceptus never has an embryo and usually presents at 8–24 weeks' gestation with PV bleeding (±the passing of grape-like tissue). The uterus may be soft, doughy and large for dates, and there may also be pre-eclampsia, hyperemesis, cardiac failure and thyrotoxicosis. USS shows a 'snowstorm appearance' and there may be multiple luteal cysts. Overall, 10% invade ('invasive mole') and the incidence of choriocarcinoma is 3%. Approximately 15% require treatment after ERPOC.

Invasive mole The mole invades the myometrium (and is therefore a histological diagnosis) and patients may present with PV bleeding weeks after an ERPOC. The possibility of invasive disease is suggested by persistently elevated serum hCG (i.e. persistent trophoblastic disease). Metastases to lung, vagina, liver, brain and the GI tract may occur, although occasionally these may regress spontaneously.

Gestational choriocarcinoma This contains both syncytiotrophoblast and cytotrophoblast and is histologically different from a hydatidiform mole (absence of villi). It may arise from a hydatidiform mole (50%) or follow an LB, SB, abortion or ectopic pregnancy. It contains maternal and paternal chromosomes unlike choriocarcinoma of ovarian origin.

Placental site trophoblastic tumour This contains largely cytotrophoblast (therefore it has lower hCG) and occurs almost exclusively following a normal pregnancy. It is much rarer than gestational choriocarcinoma and presents with amenorrhoea or irregular bleeding.

Management

Initial management

If gestational trophoblastic disease is suspected then a USS and CXR should be arranged. Blood should be sent for hCG, TFTs and 4 U of RCC crossmatched prior to undertaking the ERPOC. The risk of bleeding ±perforation is significant, but ERPOC is superior to both medical evacuation of the uterus (which may lead to increased risk of dissemination) and hysterectomy. Medical evacuation is appropriate only if a fetus (if present) is too large for surgical evacuation. It is recommended that oxytocics are avoided until after the ERPOC, and used only preoperatively to control severe haemorrhage if necessary. Mifepristone and prostaglandin analogues should also be avoided unless clinically essential.

Management after ERPOC

- Register the patient with one of the regional centres (see above).
- Monitor fortnightly hCG levels until undetectable, then monthly for 6 months and 3 monthly for the second year. The patient must wait at least 6 months from hCG=0 (or 1 year following chemotherapy) until trying for a further pregnancy. Condoms or an IUCD may be used. The COC or HRT must not be taken until the hCG has been normal for at least 6 months (to do so increases the risk of recurrence).

- Start chemotherapy if the hCG is progressively rising following the ERPOC, or is >20 000 U at 4 weeks, or if the pathology is reported as choriocarcinoma. Of those patients who develop persistent trophoblastic disease ≈80% are low risk and 20% at high risk on the scoring system shown in Table 7.6. Of the low-risk group, 80% respond to low-dose methotrexate, but 20% need additional chemotherapy because of methotrexate resistance (usually actinomycin-D and etoposide). All low-risk patients are cured. High-risk patients are usually given methotrexate and then actinomycin-D and etoposide over several cycles. If they develop drug resistance, cisplatin, cyclophosphamide and etoposide can be used. Chemotherapy is always given if the diagnosis is choriocarcinoma, or if there are metastases to the liver, brain and GI tract (80% of high-risk patients are cured).

Of long-term survivors, 85% have normal pregnancies, but if a patient has had one hydatidiform mole, the risk of a second mole is 2% and that of a third 20%. Follow-up with hCG must be undertaken after any subsequent pregnancy.

Treatment assessment
See Table 7.6.

TABLE 7.6   Prognostic factors in gestational trophoblastic disease

Score	0	1	2	4
Age	<39	>39		
Previous pregnancy	Mole	Abortion	Term pregnancy	
Interval previous pregnancy (months)	4	4–6	7–12	>12
hCG	<1000	1000–10 000	10 000–100 000	>100 000
Parental blood group		O or A	B or AB	
Size of tumour (including uterus)		3–5 cm	>5 cm	
Metastasis site		Spleen, kidney	GI, liver	Brain
No. of metastases		1–4	4–8	>8
Previous chemotherapy			Single drug	Two drugs

LEGAL ISSUES IN OBSTETRICS AND GYNAECOLOGY

Medical law and ethics are becoming increasingly important in all medical specialities, but especially in obstetrics and gynaecology. The rise in litigation in recent years has been dubbed a 'malpractice crisis'. Many obstetric claims receive large financial settlements and attract much media attention.

CONSENT

Under common law it is well recognized that every person has the right to protect their bodily integrity against invasion by others. As a general rule, medical treatment, even of a minor nature, should not proceed unless the doctor has first obtained the patient's consent. Failure to do so may constitute battery (assault in Scotland), leading to civil claims, criminal prosecution or disciplinary procedures. The only two exceptions to obtaining consent are in an emergency situation, or with an unconscious patient.

Consent may be implied (e.g. rolling up a sleeve for a blood test) or expressed (orally or in writing). What needs to be disclosed remains a topic of intense legal and ethical debate. Many patients will want to know the potential problems in great detail, others will want only the minimum of information. It might be more relevant to warn a 30-year-old obese patient seeking a hysterectomy for menstrual problems about the risks of venous thromboembolic disease, for example, than to cover excessive detail about potential bowel injury in an otherwise well 50-year-old woman with well-differentiated endometrial carcinoma going for the same operation. This would argue against general 'tick lists', although there may be a role for these in some instances (e.g. sterilization). Indeed, the issue of consent has assumed a significant place in the medical negligence debate in recent years, especially in claims for female sterilization. Some would argue that the minimum information disclosed should be the 'prudent patient' standard, i.e. what the patient thinks she should be told, whilst others argue that it should be the 'professional' standard, i.e. what the doctor thinks the patient should be told. The patient should be informed as fully as possible about the nature and consequences of treatment, and alternative therapies available, in a manner which the patient comprehends.

MEDICAL NEGLIGENCE

Although there has been a marked increase in recent years in the number of litigation claims and value of financial awards, it is still very difficult to succeed in an action of medical negligence in the UK. Not only are there practical difficulties in linking the injury of the plaintiff (or pursuer in

Scotland) to medical treatment but, in medical negligence cases, the courts still effectively allow the standard of care to be defined by the medical profession itself.

The seminal legal cases are those of Hunter vs Hanley in Scotland [Hunter vs Hanley 1955 SC 200] and the English case of Bolam [Bolam vs Friern Hospital Management Committee [1957] 2 All ER 118, [1957] 1 WLR 582.], both of which define the essence of medical negligence. The Bolam dictum states, 'a doctor is not negligent if he acts in accordance with a practice accepted at the time as proper by a responsible body of medical opinion'. This is applicable not only to diagnosis and treatment but also the giving of information.

If a patient suffers harm as a result of treatment in hospital she may bring action for damages against the hospital. Vicarious liability means that the trust is liable for any errors made by the doctor in the course of his or her employment.

For an action of medical negligence to succeed the patient must be able to show three things:

- the doctor owed the patient a duty of care,
- the doctor was in breach of that duty (i.e. failed to provide care of an adequate standard),
- the patient suffered harm as a consequence of that breach.

The burden of proof lies with the patient pursuing a claim of negligence. It is for the patient to show that, on the balance of probabilities, the doctor failed to meet the standard of care expected.

CONFIDENTIALITY

The requirement to protect patient confidentiality has long been included in the ethical codes of healthcare professionals (e.g. the hippocratic oath). Protecting patient confidentiality may give rise to some very difficult moral and legal dilemmas (e.g. young girls requesting contraception, HIV testing in pregnancy).

There are exceptions to the confidentiality rule (General Medical Council, 1995). These include emergency situations, if the health or safety of the others are placed at serious risk, or if it is felt to be in the patient's best interests for confidentiality to be breached. Patients should always be told before confidentiality is breached.

FETO-MATERNAL CONFLICT

Modern technology such as ultrasound scanning, which permits visualization of the fetus in utero, has led many to view the fetus as a person and patient, separate from the pregnant woman. This may create feto-maternal conflict, when the interests of the mother appear to diverge from those of the fetus.

Recent cases of court-authorized caesarean sections have highlighted the difficulties faced by doctors when a pregnant woman refuses to accept treatment which is thought by medical staff to be in the best interests of either herself or her baby. These judgments from the High Court which sanctioned the performance of caesarean sections against the mother's wishes received strong criticism for two main reasons.

- They contradict the generally held principle of the right to self-determination (autonomy). Many legal cases have demonstrated that, provided a patient has sufficient mental capability to understand the treatment options available they have the right to refuse treatment, even if it endangers their own life.
- It has been established in both the civil and criminal law that the fetus is not a person with legal rights and, as such, the courts do not have the power to protect the fetus.

The Court of Appeal subsequently reviewed these cases and concluded that it is unlawful to perform a caesarean section against a woman's wishes, if she is mentally competent. It is recommended that problem cases should be identified and brought before the courts early. There should be evidence, preferably from a psychiatrist, as to the woman's background and her mental capacity, and she should be legally represented in court. Doctors are under a duty to respect an advanced directive (i.e. expressed in advance of the emergency) from a competent patient refusing consent (e.g. one cannot perform a caesarean section against the patient's wishes if an advanced directive has been given against caesarean).

IF SOMETHING GOES WRONG

Most procedures carry recognized complications, despite being carried out by the most skilful and experienced operator. If complications arise they should be taken seriously, appropriately managed and the patient and relatives should be fully informed. Advice from senior colleagues should be sought at an early stage. Even if it is felt that an error has been made by somebody else, it is unwise to criticise another healthcare professional in front of the patient, particularly if the full facts are not yet known. However, if a mistake has been made, it is good practice to admit it and apologise to the patient personally. This does not imply negligence. Indeed, failure to disclose the error, provide information, and offer an apology increase the risk of litigation (Lancet 1994;343:1609).

Medicine can never be free of mishaps. In our current medical culture, in which 'error' is often equated with 'incompetence', admission of errors to patients or fellow professionals is difficult. However, with clinical governance becoming an increasingly important aspect of healthcare, it is essential that mistakes are acknowledged and lessons learnt to prevent avoidable errors occurring again. Nobody is perfect, and not everybody owns a retrospectoscope.

BPD (mm)	Gestation (weeks)
18	12+1
19	12+3
20	12+4
21	12+6
22	13+1
23	13+2
24	13+4
25	13+6
26	14+1
27	14+3
28	14+5
29	14
32	15
35	16
38	17
42	18
46	19
49	20
52	21
55	22

BPD (mm)	Gestation (weeks)
58	23
61	24
64	25
68	26
71	27
74	28
77	29
80	30
83	31
85	32
87	33
89	34
91	35
92	36
94	37
95	38
96	39
97	40
98	41
99	42

Appendix I Bi-parietal diameter.

CRL (mm)	– 2 SD	Gestation (weeks)	+ 2 SD
6	6 + 1	7 + 1	8 + 0
7	6 + 3	7 + 2	8 + 2
8	6 + 4	7 + 4	8 + 3
9	6 + 6	7 + 6	8 + 6
10	7 + 1	8 + 0	9 + 0
11	7 + 2	8 + 2	9 + 1
12	7 + 3	8 + 3	9 + 3
13	7 + 5	8 + 4	9 + 4
14	7 + 6	8 + 6	9 + 6
15	8 + 0	9 + 0	10 + 0
16	8 + 2	9 + 2	10 + 1
17	8 + 3	9 + 3	10 + 2
18	8 + 4	9 + 4	10 + 4
19	8 + 5	9 + 5	10 + 5
20	8 + 6	9 + 6	10 + 6
21	9 + 0	10 + 0	11 + 0
22	9 + 1	10 + 1	11 + 1
23	9 + 2	10 + 2	11 + 2
24	9 + 3	10 + 3	11 + 3
26	9 + 5	10 + 5	11 + 5
28	9 + 6	11 + 0	12 + 1
30	10 + 1	11 + 2	12 + 2
32	10 + 2	11 + 3	12 + 4
34	10 + 4	11 + 5	12 + 5
36	10 + 5	11 + 6	13 + 0
38	10 + 6	12 + 1	13 + 2
40	11 + 1	12 + 2	13 + 3
42	11 + 2	12 + 3	13 + 4
44	11 + 3	12 + 4	13 + 6
46	11 + 5	12 + 6	14 + 0
48	11 + 6	13 + 0	14 + 2
50	11 + 6	13 + 1	14 + 3

Appendix 2 Crown–rump length (CRL).

Gestation from LMP (weeks)	Approx. sac on TV scan diameter (mm)	Earliest findings on TV scan	Earliest findings on TA scan
5	5	Sac	
5.5	8	FH and fetal pole	Sac
6	13		
6.5	17		FH and fetal pole
7	23		
8	32		
9	40		

Appendix 3 First trimester USS findings (experienced ultrasonographers).

BI-PARIETAL DIAMETER
5th, 50th and 95th centiles

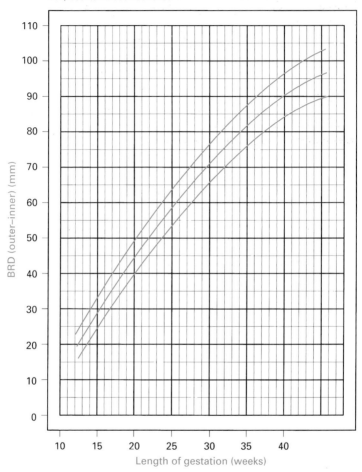

Appendix 4 Bi-parietal diameter: 5th, 50th and 95th centiles.

ABDOMINAL CIRCUMFERENCE
5th, 50th and 95th centiles

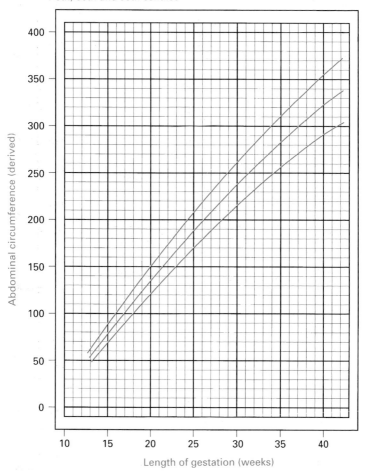

Appendix 5 Abdominal circumference: 5th, 50th and 95th centiles.

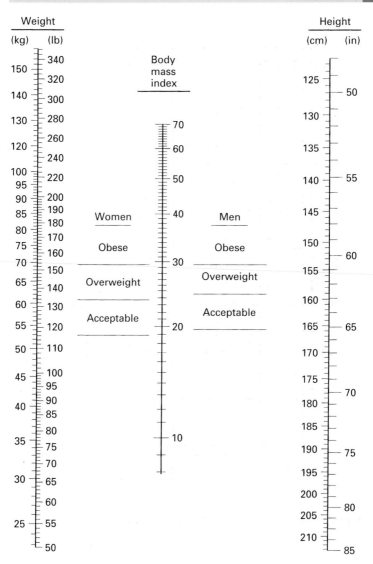

Appendix 6 Body mass index.

INDEX